Reclaim Your Life

Your Guide to Aid
Healing of Endometriosis

By
Carolyn Levett

The publication of this book is supported by
www.endo-resolved.com

The motivational advice website for women and girls
who suffer from the disabling disease of Endometriosis

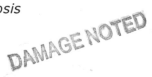

Second Edition 2008 by www-endo-resolved.com

Author Carolyn Levett
Copyright © Endo Resolved

ISBN 978-0-9556785-1-6

Disclaimer:

The advice in this book is intended solely for informational and educational purposes only and not as medical advice. Please consult a medical professional if you have questions about your health.

Dedication

This book is dedicated to all the women and girls in the world who suffer from the disabling disease of endometriosis. Their many stories of pain, suffering and distress led to the writing of this book – to give others hope and encouragement that they too could achieve healing from this dreadful disease.

iv

Contents

Introduction

Part One

Part Two

Part Three

Part Four

About the Author

Carolyn Levett is the website owner of www.endo-resolved.com which she put together to provide positive advice and support for women and girls suffering from endometriosis. She was diagnosed herself with severe endometriosis and decided to follow her own path to healing using homeopathy, supplements, diet, and lots of determination. After 4 years of healing, a second laparoscopy confirmed that she was indeed free of endometriosis.

She spent the early part of her life in rural Sussex in England, living with her Father and brother under difficult family circumstances. Over the years she has studied and practised many subjects in her life to include a BA in the Arts, Interior Design, Textile Art, Community Development, small business management, Aromatherapy, Massage, Herbalism, African Drumming and Samba, Horse Riding, organic gardening, and continues to learn new things every day. She is currently living and working in Andalucia, Spain with her partner running a business in Painting Holidays.

Introduction

This book is for women everywhere, who are looking for hope, inspiration, and confidence that they can achieve relief from the distressing disease called Endometriosis. This is your antidote against all the negative information you may have heard or read, about your long-term prospects of dealing with this disease. Time and time again you have been told that endometriosis is 'not curable'.

What is a 'cure' anyway? The word 'cure' is very loaded with expectations and assumptions. What I am saying is that you have the power and possibilities to improve your health to such an extent, as to eliminate your symptoms; to go into remission; to feel healthy, vital and disease-free; restore your health; rectify the imbalances in your body - how else can I put it - to eliminate the disease and reclaim your life.

I was told by my gynaecologist that I had one of the worst cases of endometriosis she had seen and that I was in a complete mess internally. Her prognosis was not good at all. Her suggested method of treatment was just as bad. I reeled with shock at first, but I soon gathered my energies, found out my options, collected information about the disease and gradually found my own path towards the goal of healing myself. It was not a quick fix; repairing and healing the body takes time, patience, commitment and faith.

I have remained totally free of endometriosis for many years. The certainty that I was free of this disease comes from the evidence I was given after my second Laparoscopy, but you will read all this soon.

It has taken a while to arrive at a time in my life where I was given space and opportunity to be able to write this book. The aims and objectives behind this book came about gradually. Endometriosis has been history for me for many years now, and I have been able to pick up the pieces of my life and move forward. It was not until I obtained my first computer with Internet access some years ago, that this idea started to develop.

When I first starting using the Internet I was reading up on everything from gardening to gismos. I then started to come across websites about endometriosis, and was astounded by the amount of information now available. I was also astounded to read time and time again that endometriosis is absolutely incurable. It disturbed me to think of all those women who were searching for information, solutions, and hope, only to be told over and over that there is 'no cure' for this disease.

I wanted to put this straight. To redress the balance of negative information. How was it that I had healed! - and yet millions of women today are told that there is no hope of any permanent solutions, no long-term successful treatment, and no hope of a cure. So the impetus and birth of this book came about from my own feelings of anger at the definitive statements saying there was 'no cure for Endometriosis'; and my feelings of concern for all those millions of women who are left feeling hopeless and desperate.

This book is aimed purely at the women who have this disease. It is not aimed at the medical profession - although it would help them to read it - or the hundreds of researchers who are searching desperately for treatments as well as causes.

This book is not written by yet another medical professional who has their own 'view' on this disease. It is not another book about 'coping strategies'. It is not another book full of complex medical information.

This book is written by a woman who had the disease, conquered the disease, and now wants to pass on as much positive and useful information, ideas, support and energy as possible.

I spent many months researching the subject of endometriosis from many different angles before I started writing. As well as my own experience with endometriosis, I needed to understand the subject with a clear over-view. I wanted to put this disease into context. I wanted to understand the how, why, where, when and to whom this was happening to. I am not a medical professional, researcher, or journalist, just an ordinary human being. I have no special inherent talents, no far-out healing abilities. I am just like any other woman, and I enforce this issue over and over again in this book.

I apologise in advance if my grammar is not totally accurate in places, but I have tried to write this book in certain places as though I am talking to you in person. I felt this approach would be more user-friendly and encouraging. I also tried my utmost to be accurate with the medical facts of this disease. Mind you there are not many absolute facts surrounding endometriosis; what we do have is lots of speculation and statistics.

The contents of this book are written with full integrity on my part; not to mislead anyone, not to give false hope. But I am adamant that the possibilities and outcomes suggested here are totally valid and it is completely within the grasp of women to radically improve their health and even to heal themselves of endometriosis.

Yours with healing thoughts

Carolyn Levett
Endo Resolved
www.endo-resolved.com

Part One
My Personal Story

My Personal Story

Finding out that you have a real illness, a disease, something that isn't going to clear up in a few weeks or months is like opening a door and on the other side is a huge black chasm, and you fall into that chasm. And you keep falling.......... the more you find out, the further you fall. Then later, when it dawns on you all the ways this illness is going to affect your entire life, you realise that you have not hit the bottom of the chasm yet. What else is going to hit you! What else does this entail! What does this all mean! Why has this happened! What have I done wrong to my body? I do not deserve this. This happens to other people.

This is my story of a fight to get back to the light and out of the chasm. It has been a long chapter in my life and one that has shaped me, reshaped me, and made me tougher, stronger and so much wiser. There is a positive end to this story and I am writing it mostly to provide help, support and inspiration to other women (as well as their partners), and I am also writing it as a final cleansing of my own soul. Like a symbolic 'full stop' to that part of my life.

Early Signs

After finalising my arts degree in the late 80's I spent 3 years working voluntarily on an arts project with 2 other graduates to set up an open access arts workshop facility. Unfortunately this project never came to full fruition due to lack of funding, so the project was wound up. (Now there is an interesting turn of phrase, using the words 'wound up', considering the subject I am covering here, and how that seems to be a metaphor for the wound-up sensation of this illness).

During the last year that I worked on the project I started to feel generally run down and was prone to catch colds and any other bugs going around. I was working very hard on the project with lots of important meetings, funding applications, paper work, reports, devising the project and so on. All this work was being done on a voluntary basis, with no prospect of any salary on the horizon. We were working hard to try and resolve this through funding, but it just was not happening. I then caught gastro-enteritis and I had it very bad. I hardly ate anything for nearly 2 weeks and it took me a long time to get over it. It was soon after this that the arts project was finished.

Around this time I started to get other niggling symptoms with abdominal pain and problems with my periods. Then a few months later, after a very emotional upset with the break-up of a relationship I became very low. My symptoms worsened over the course of the next few months - I seemed to go down hill very fast. I started to feel very run down, very fluish, more abdominal pain, very painful periods, and intestinal upsets, gum infections, sleep problems. At first my doctor diagnosed it as Pelvic Inflammatory Disease (in the gums!!!!), prescribed 2 courses of anti-biotics, but I was not getting any better.

After much persistence on my part I asked to be referred to a gynaecologist at the local hospital. I knew that all my problems related to a gynaecological malfunction of some sort. I had done some reading to see what it could be, but was none the wiser. My hospital appointment took a few months to come through. But eventually I got to see the gynaecologist, and I told her of all my symptoms. The gynaecologist could not give me any concrete ideas or even any clues as to what was wrong with me so a laparoscopy was suggested, to investigate what was going on. She described what a laparoscopy was, how the operation was performed, and what she hoped to achieve from the operation. She explained that the main function of the operation was to get a diagnosis for all the symptoms I was suffering.

I had never had an operation in my life. I was as worried about the actual operation and the anaesthetic as I was about finding out what was wrong with me. I had never had any of the childhood operations like having my tonsils taken out or appendix taken out. I had not even had any stitches, no broken bones, nothing. This was my first introduction to hospital life.

My operation was scheduled for 2 weeks before Christmas. The hospital was very old and grey and menacing in its appearance. The staff were all very matter of fact in their manner. To get from the ward to the operating theatre patients had to be wheeled outside from one building to another. On the morning of my operation it was grey and raining. I was given a pre-med, covered in blankets to keep me warm, and I was wheeled to the main door of the ward. An umbrella was used to keep me sheltered from the rain whilst we took the journey across the hospital complex. I cannot remember much more of my very first journey to the operating theatre because of the pre-med, and I was very drowsy.

I came round from the operation later that day feeling groggy, sick and depressed. The staff nurse came to see me and said that I could go home the next day and she would also give me the date to come back and talk to the gynaecologist. I lay there thinking that this situation was just awful. Do they do this to all people. Open them up and tell them to come back in a few weeks before they find out what was discovered and how the operation went.

The next day I packed my few belongings, was given a date just after Christmas to come back to see the gynaecologist and went home. I had got most things ready for Christmas before I went into hospital, and my partner at the time organised the last few bits and pieces. We got my flat looking lovely and festive and had plenty of logs for the stove. I decided to try and enjoy Christmas and not to focus on my recent experience or to start chewing over what was wrong with me. In fact I was rather optimistic. After reading about different gynaecological disorders I had narrowed it down to a few common ailments I thought it could be; something that could be treated with a simple operation. Little did I know.........

Diagnosis

When I went back to the gynaecologist 3 weeks after the operation she said I had endometriosis, my reproductive organs were in such a mess with cysts all over my abdominal cavity, adhesions and scar tissue, that I really should have a total hysterectomy. But as I was considering having children, and being only in my twenties, then she would put me on a course of drug treatment to try and clear some of the active endometriosis. She would then operate again later to 'tidy up the damage left behind'.

I tried to take in what she was saying. I tried to stay focused. I tried to enter into a dialogue with her. To have a meaningful conversation. Tried to get to grips with what she was saying. Tried to understand the consequences of this information. I went hot with anxiety. Then I went cold with fear. I then just went numb. Cysts..... adhesions..... organs stuck together..... infertility..... not curable..... male hormone drug treatment..... more surgery..... hysterectomy..... in a complete mess..... one of the worst cases of endometriosis I have seen..... that's me she is talking about..... is it..... No..... it can't be that serious..... I can still walk, talk, go to work..... what the hell is she on about.........

I was given another 2 weeks by my gynaecologist to go away and think about things, then to return to see her to discuss the start of treatment. My head was spinning to put it very mildly. My numb state continued for another few days. I could not talk to anyone. Then friends started to find out how things had gone. They started to ring up. Started to call round. Started to give me advice. Started to shake me out of my numb shocked state.

My network of women friends were very supportive. Most of these women were astute and politically aware individuals. During my time at college I too had learnt to become more assertive, to ask questions and not to take things on face value. For this reason, I now started to hunt for any information I could relating to the bombshell that had been dropped on me. My friends also helped in whatever way they could; by putting me in touch with organisations, by lending me books, and by simply being there to listen.

I found out that the drug treatment being offered to me acts like a male hormone, which when taken by women acts on the system to induce a pseudo menopause, stops the menstrual cycle and in turn is supposed to give the reproductive organs a rest from the monthly cycle, so that the internal damage can subside. The drug being offered was Danazol.

I found this information initially from the literature sent by the Endometriosis Society based in London, and I also found the contact for my local endometriosis support group. So I rang up and found the time and place of their next meeting.

It was now late winter as I headed off to my first meeting with the endometriosis support group, which was held at a community centre in town. Most of these women were in their 30's with varying stages of the illness. I very soon found out that most of the women in the group were taking a drug treatment like Danazol or similar, to put them in a pseudo-menopause, which was the same drug that my gynaecologist wanted me to use. I asked these women how they were coping with it. Most of them were having a horrific time - depression, weight gain, nausea, muscle cramps, constant hunger, greasy hair, headaches, and dizziness. My God I thought, I REALLY do not think I want to go down that path, to put my body through all that. What would the long term effects be, what other side effects are there that are not know about.

Having found out more details of the drug treatment being offered, I vowed never to return to the gynaecologist if that was the only option on offer. When talking to the other women at the endometriosis support group about their experiences of taking the drug treatment route, I was appalled. I was appalled by what the drugs did and appalled by what these women had to go through. The side effects of the drugs sounded worse than the endometriosis. Not all women suffer these effects, but I did not want to find out what it would do to me. I knew in my gut that this form of drug treatment was totally wrong for me. Alarm bells went off in my head. I seemed to know intuitively that I would become very ill with the side effects; and would it cure the endometriosis, NO. It just comes back as soon as you stop taking it. O.K., the idea was to get respite from the normal monthly cycle of active endometriosis getting worse and worse, and then have an operation to get 'cleared up', but I felt I was entering a mine field of damaging, invasive drug and knife therapy. None of what I had been told seemed to be leading towards long term healing; to regain my health.

Journey of Self Help

From that point on I decided to go down the path of self-help. I gathered as much information as I could from the Endometriosis Society, from the library and from talking to other women. My God, it is so different now. There was limited advice on the Internet back then..... imagine it. There is an abundance of information on the Internet today about endometriosis (possibly too much). If you do a search for endometriosis at Google you will get hundreds of thousands of results. That is a hell of a lot of information.

But back when I was diagnosed the Internet was still quite new and most of us could not afford computers. Finding information had to be done the old fashioned way. But I needed to get informed. I searched for as much advice I could get my hands on about self help measures, what the causes of the disease are, and most importantly, I scoured around everywhere for any 'how I got better stories'.

Not just getting well from endometriosis, but getting well from other serious diseases as well. I needed motivation, I needed guidance, and I needed support. I needed solid, positive affirmations that people can heal from even the most impossible cases of ill health. I knew that stories like this existed, and I rooted around for them in earnest.

I knew I had a fight on my hands. No, it was more than that it was a long battle. I had secured a job in the meantime and was working full time at this point, and coping the best I could, but I was having many days off sick from work. My energy levels were on the floor; I had chronic sleep problems, bowel problems and the pain and fatigue got worse and worse. I got to the point where I could only walk a few hundred yards because of the pain in my abdomen and groin.

I started in earnest taking the vitamin and herbal supplements recommended by the Endometriosis Society. I was also reading all I could about health, nutrition and alternative therapies. Remember, there was limited Internet information available at this time, so I had to do all my research the hard way; by going to the library, sending for information leaflets published by the Endometriosis Society (and having to pay for them), and by buying books at alternative book stores. It was a very slow, drawn out process.

Around this time I decided to try some counselling, to help me deal with some of the emotional stuff I was dealing with, and to have someone to talk to who could be objective. My councillor was a lovely caring young man, who was himself going through counselling because of his own ill health. He was able to make very astute observations about my mannerisms, my body language and how my body was functioning. During one session he laid his hands on my abdomen whilst I was lying down and he could tell that I had eaten my lunch whilst I was stood up, which he said was not good for me. Unfortunately I could not continue with the counselling, as I could not afford to pay for that as well as all the other costs that were adding up. Going for counselling can be quite expensive and I needed to use any spare money for tangible health support measures like the diet supplements.

I then attended a basic herbal medicine course where the fees were subsidised. I did enjoy the course but herbal medicine did not feel like the correct course of action to deal with my endometriosis. Not that I would have self-treated with herbalism, but I wanted an insight into this topic. After a few months of floundering, trying different things, reading further about different therapies, I finally gravitated towards Homeopathy and went in search for a Homeopath.

I had done some general reading on the subject of alternative medicine, healing, counselling, and different therapies. One piece of advice I took note of, was not to start collecting therapists or trying too many different therapies. Your body will not know what is working and what is not. You can start clutching at straws. You will not get the benefits of any given therapy. My decision to go for Homeopathy was a purely gut feeling. There was no logical reasoning; it just 'felt' right.

A friend recommended a Homeopath to me; I was given her phone number, and I rang and made an initial appointment. One of the most important things about working with a therapist, alternative practitioner or your own doctor for that matter is to feel that you can trust that person and feel at ease with them. As soon as I met Julia I knew I was in good hands and I liked her. After our first session I knew I was in the right place, following the correct course of action for me.

I had read during my research that other women had had great success in treating, relieving or even 'curing' their endometriosis using herbalism, acupuncture, diet, yoga or homeopathy. We all seem to gravitate naturally to what is right for us eventually, and homeopathy was right for me. I knew it intuitively.

It was now a year after I began to feel really ill, and I began what was to be a 4-year course of healing with my homeopath. There were many layers of healing and repair work to do; years of damage to repair. Not only does homeopathy work on the physical body, it also works on the emotional level.

As well as working on my endometriosis, we also worked on issues around my childhood and any past illnesses. Homeopathy, like other Alternative Therapies treats the whole person, not just the symptoms. This is where so much of modern medicine goes wrong. Doctors give out drugs to alleviate the symptoms, but they do not get at the root cause. The initial problem IS STILL THERE. I grant that many drugs do help people cope better with whatever illness they have, but that is all. Sometimes the side effects of such drugs can be awful, if not worse than the illness itself. There are no ill effects with homeopathy. Even if you are given the wrong remedy, because it will just bypass your system as not being relevant or needed.

Julia, my homeopath, was very astute at dream interpretation, and a lot of work was done around my dreams and their sub-conscious meaning. Our dreams can speak volumes about how we are feeling, and what is happening to our bodies at a cellular level. We all need to listen to our bodies a lot more. That is why we get cravings for certain foods, because we have a shortage in our diet somewhere.

I went to see Julia about every 4 to 6 weeks at first. I took a variety of homeopathic remedies, each one dealing with a different aspect of my healing. The remedies were given in different strengths depending on what was needed to 'shift' at that time. One of the remedies I took had been diluted to the millionth strength, which means that the active ingredients remaining in that remedy are microscopic, in fact almost non-existent. This is where homeopathy really starts to enter the realms of quantum physics. The word quantum coming from the Latin for 'how much'! But with homeopathy, the more a remedy is 'diluted' the stronger it becomes. This is why many doctors and scientists find it impossible to come to terms with any theories as to how homeopathy works. They do not believe it is possible to have any effect on the body at such minute doses.

Healing in Context

At first there was a slow and gradual improvement to my health, but it was very slow. There were so many problems to deal with; so many layers of healing to do. When I went to see Julia, our consultation sessions would last for about an hour. She would ask me many questions about my general well-being and how I felt I was doing. She would always ask me if there were any changes in my life or if I had noticed any changes taking place within me.

We would cover many subjects around my well-being, my body and what it was doing, what my mind-set was like, any dreams I was having and other subjects that would not seem relevant to me, but they would to a homeopath. Julia would usually send me my next homeopathic remedy in the post a few days later so that she had time to absorb what had been said, and she could decide on the next relevant remedy for me. I asked her not to write on the packet what the remedy was so that I would not go and look it up and then start puzzling why she had given me that particular remedy.

Like I said earlier, I was working full time now, having found work after winding up the arts workshop project. But my heart was not in my work, partly because it was a temporary contract working in a subject far removed from that of an Arts Degree Graduate. I was working in Economic Development at the local Chamber of Commerce, for a separate government initiative, the Enterprise Agency. I got the job by default because I and the other graduates had done small business training in order to secure the capital funding for the project. Despite my lack of interest in my job, I had a reasonable wage coming in now, which helped to pay for my homeopathic consultation sessions, my diet supplements and vitamins, and kept body and soul together.

As my financial situation had improved, and I was starting to pick up a bit health wise, I decided to go to the States to see and old friend from college who was now living there. I decided to go for the whole month of February, just when the weather in the UK is at its worst, and it would also coincide with my birthday. The trip did me a lot of good and I came home feeling very positive and energised.

Soon after getting home again I decided it was time I looked for another job in earnest. I HATE JOB HUNTING. But it had to be done. I hate job-hunting so much, because it is one of those activities in life where you are not in charge of your own destiny. The whole shape of your future life rests completely in the hands of others - yes, you can decide which jobs to apply for, but that is as far as your power and self-definition goes. The economic climate in the UK was dire at this time, with many people being made redundant, and the competition for jobs was fierce. But I battled on. I did try very hard to obtain work in the arts but it was a closed shop. The only way to get a good job was to know 'someone on the inside'. The classic situation of not what you know but who you know.

I applied for lots of jobs and was getting nowhere except more and more disillusioned. This had a knock on effect with my health and I started to feel ill again. The respite and benefits I achieved from my holiday started to disappear. But I had to continue. I had to pay the rent, to pay the bills and all that other stuff of modern day life. All I wanted to do was run away from it all really. I just wanted to be well, to pack a small bag and go off into the blue yonder. I was beginning to feel I had had a belly full of everything. Then at the eleventh hour I secured another job, but yes I was still stuck (there is that metaphor again) in the field of Economic Development. But this time I was in the Local Authority, so I reckoned on good job security here. How wrong I was .... why does life keep dishing out the joker of the pack just for me?

The job turned out to be a political minefield. Yes, I was working in local government which by default is political, but I was working in the most volatile area of local government, being economic development. In the space of 18 months I had 4 job descriptions, 3 line-managers and had moved office 3 times. The issue of my changing job description had the worst effect on me.

You may be wondering why am I going into such detail here about the pitfalls of my career. It is because we are all the sum total of our parts. We are all a reflection of our experiences. These experiences were affecting me deeply. They were affecting my well being at a fundamental level.

Back to the issue of my changing job description though. My original job description, and the reason I had applied for the job in the first place, was suddenly thrown out of the window when there was a change in political power at local government level. I had spent about 10 months working with community groups in the city, getting to know people in the community, building their trust, as I was the broker between them and the powers that be. We were working on community based economic development ideas, like furniture recycling stores, skills training for unemployed people, community nurseries. Some really good viable ideas and pilot projects were devised and some of these ideas were beginning to take shape.

Then the plug was pulled, not only on me but all the groups I had been working with. With the change in political power from left to right, I now had to work on mainstream, hard-core economic development stuff - small business start up advice, and act like a minion in the Enterprise Centre. I HATED IT. I had clashes with my new line manager, I hated the toxic environment in the newly merged department and I went home many nights in tears.

My inner resolve could not tolerate the huge impact on my life that my job was having. I had to get out. I had to leave a secure job with good holiday entitlements, annual pay increases and long term security, because the rules had totally changed. The final crunch came when I was told to go and see the head of the Economic Development Unit for a dressing down. **This was official**, but what the hell had I done. I arrived in the 'big cheeses' office to be told

1 I am taking too much time off sick
2 I have an attitude problem
3 Not to air my views so much

I went home that night and got copiously drunk!

After 18 months in this job, my job hunt was on again - in earnest. I was looking for something with similar pay but fewer hours now. Working full time was too much for me.

A Roof over my Head

As I had secured the job at the Local Authority with what I thought were good long-term prospects, I had obtained my first mortgage and bought myself a small house. This is another saga in itself which needs to be described, to fill in all the pieces of my puzzle. When I look back now I wonder how the hell I ever managed to get over endometriosis with all the stress I had in my life. So I will continue.

When I was first diagnosed with endometriosis I was living in rented accommodation. I had my own flat which was a conversion in a big old sprawling house on the outskirts of the city. The house was so big it accommodated 8 self-contained flats, and its own sprawling grounds surrounded it. The house had a lot of history and was built in the early 19th century, originally built for a rich local businessman.

The house maintained many of its original features including the sweeping staircase, with views vaulting right up to the roof which had stained glass skylight windows. In its hey day the house had servant quarters, tennis court and landscaped gardens. It was rumoured that Gracie Fields stayed there at one time. During the war the house had been used as a 'gentleman's' club', otherwise known as a brothel. There was still some decorative evidence of this, with one entire wall in Elaine's' flat downstairs covered in mirrors.

The conversion to flats took place soon after the war, and the standard and style of the fitments of the flats was testament to this. The sink in my kitchen was an old stone sink with a wooden draining board and an old gas cooker dating back to the 40's. The main living rooms in the house were huge and kept to their original size. Trying to heat these spaces was a nightmare and after my first winter there I installed a log-burning stove.

The property was 'In Trust', so the rent was very cheap. All the tenants mixed well and it was a good supportive little community. Of course the grounds were now overrun with brambles and shrubs, but collectively we looked after the garden area closest to the house. One of the benefits of living at this house was that pets were allowed. I had moved here from a small first floor flat with my 1 year old Border Collie. As soon as she saw the garden she thought all her birthdays had come at once. She also got on very well with Elaine's dog Max, and they used to hurtle around the garden together for hours on end.

I had been living there for just over 2 years, when one day we all received the news that was to force all of us to change our lives. The property was to be sold to property developers. There was no compensation to be had. We did have the option to look for temporary accommodation and move back in once the house had been revamped. But we all knew that the rent would probably go up by at least 300%. We were all given 4 months notice to quit.

I had been very happy living at the house with its community of like-minded people and now I was forced again to make a huge upheaval in my life. I really did not need this. I was still working at the Local Authority at this point, and the job was still going fine at this time. This was when I decided it was time to think about buying a place of my own. The other people in the house were all doing the same.

But this was one of the worse times to buy a house in the UK as the housing market was going mad. I mean absolutely 'pear-shaped'. House prices were 'going through the roof'. You could go to an Estate Agent to enquire about a property, which may have only been on the market for only a few days, only to find that it had sold ……….. and someone had paid more than the asking price. It was a nightmare.

It was summer time now. I was travelling round most evenings after work looking for the 'For Sale' signs outside houses, and then ringing Estate Agents first thing the next morning. I was told the same thing over and over again. 'Sorry that one had been sold!' Because of my limited budget I could only enquire about houses at the lower price range. Of course houses in this price range were selling very fast. People were desperate not to be left out of the housing market. I was having to look further and further a field in my hunt for a home. The ethics/ economics of house ownership in the UK is almost immoral. To have a roof over your head is a basic human need and right in our modern day society, but to purchase a basic simple home requires the average worker to commit 25 to 30 years of their life, committing on average 60% of their income to pay for it. Is life meant to be this tough? Why is society designed like this? I will stop there before I go off on a social/political crusade!

My new partner was giving me a lot of support through all this upheaval. He too had lived at the big house, and he had since purchased a tiny cottage on the outskirts of the city. I had the offer to move in with him, but firstly I did not want to have to move in with him by default, and secondly, I did not want to move to a building site, as there was a lot of work to do on his house. So he accompanied me on my house hunting trips to give me advice and help keep my spirits up.

I was still seeing Julia, on a very regular basis. I need more support than ever from my homeopathy to help me keep going during this time. Of course, whenever I had my period every thing just had to stop. I felt too awful to do anything. The pains in my abdomen were crippling. I was also starting to feel generally very run down all the time, as though I had the flu. I had to take 2/3 days off work every time I had my period. I was also starting to have difficulty in walking too far. I would get deep, dragging pains in my abdomen and down into the top of my legs.

I remember one particular day earlier in the summer, before all the issue of being forced to move had reared its head. It was a pleasant spring day and the sun was shining. I was sat on my window seat looking over the view. In the far distance the open moorland could be seen beyond the edge of the city. I was desperate to get out for a good long walk with my dog. Somewhere open and wild. But I just did not have the stamina in the last few months to do this. As I sat there looking at the view, I noticed an area of green open land. It was on the other side of the valley about half a mile away. It was too steep to build houses on, so it had been left as an open grassy area. I calculated that it would only be about 15 minutes walk away from where I sat.

So I set off with Charcoal, my dog. I did not walk too fast so that I did not tire. I just went at a nice leisurely pace. I got to the bottom of the hill, crossed the main road, worked my way through the houses and got closer to the green slope. I was starting to flag; my legs were beginning to get very heavy. But I decided to continue and take it very steady. Eventually, I reached the bottom of the open green area. The slope rose up rather steeply. More steeply than I had anticipated.

After about 25 minutes of walking I started to feel like an old lady of 90. But I had reached that stubborn, determined point to achieve what I had set out to do. I mean, why the hell could I not walk up a grass slope after only 25 minutes walking at the my young age. This was ridiculous.

I started in vain hope up the slope. Every step got harder and harder. I was pushing my hands on my thighs to act as additional leverage. It was like swimming in treacle. I started to feel my head go light. I could hear the blood rushing through my ears. I felt sick. Then I started to feel as though I would black out. I stopped and looked round. I had managed to walk about 50 yards up the slope, but I could not walk any further.

I sat down on the grass and just sobbed. Charcoal, my dog came and sat next to me. She leaned against me as if she knew what was going on and what I was feeling. We sat there for about half an hour. And I just sobbed. This was the time in my life when things should be taking off. I had done my degree; I had gained lots of experience with the arts project. I was in my late 20's. My career should be lifting off now, I should start to think about growing up, buying a house, settling down with someone, having kids.

My life had included the student bit, the late nights, and the mad life of youth. I had done the dropout bit before that. I had done the rebellious bit before that. I had done the leaving home early bit.

It was now time to start shaping up my life and making grown up plans. So here I was sat on the grass in the middle of the day, crying my eyes out and unable to use my body. It had stopped bloody working.

And on top of that I kept having all this shit thrown at me with normal practical things in life just going completely haywire. None of it, absolutely none of it was my fault.

It was around this time that I was having horrendous nightmares. The sort of nightmares that make you wake up very suddenly, full of fear and anxiety. I would have these nightmares night after night.

I was going through a period of dealing with a lot of buried wounds and emotional damage from my past, which was being brought to the surface by the homeopathy. I was remembering and trying to come to terms with old wounds from my childhood, of being dumped by my mother in a children's home along with my brother at the age of 4. I was remembering the foster homes, the temporary stay with my mother, the court orders and then being reunited with my brother and father 2 years later.

I was also remembering with anger the experiences of myself and my brother being looked after by an ageing 'Victorian' type housekeeper, who would hit us all the time; hit us for asking the wrong things, hit us for not asking permission to go to the toilet, hit us for being 2 minutes late for anything, hit us for crying and hit us for just existing. All this was unknown to my father, and small kids do not say anything when they are frightened for fear of reprisals. So we just kept quiet, very quiet and looked to each other for support.

All this pain had to come out because it had not up to this point. Even writing these details now is still painful but it is also therapeutic. The more we express our feelings, the less the anger and pain is bottled up and the less it will fester causing further damage to the body and soul.

So the bad dreams and nightmares I was having were partly related to my past and obviously strongly related to my present. Some nights I woke up in a state of 'primal scream'. One night all this pain became unbearable and as I lay in my bed in the dark, with my thoughts and emotions crashing around internally like a violent storm, there was a sudden loud **BANG** inside my head and my head jolted forward violently. I found out later that what I had experienced was similar to an epileptic fit. All the synapses in my brain fired off at once, like a safety valve, as my soul could not cope with the stress and pain any more. I had had a complete mental meltdown. My emotions were simply shot to pieces.

The nightmares went on for months and they would shake my emotions to the core and I would wake up and cry - hard, very hard, for all the pain. The pain of getting ill, the physical pain, the pain of possibly being infertile, the pain of loosing a grip on my career, the pain of loosing my social life, of loosing my sex life, the pain of not being able to lead a normal life, the pain of my past, the pain of my present, the fear of my future. There was absolutely no colour in my life. This was one of the lowest points during my illness, but it was also a very important part of my healing process. I had let a lot of emotional baggage come out.

Then the bad dreams and nightmares subsided. I now started to have fits of anger instead. I started throwing crockery around. I WAS ANGRY. I felt every justification to show my bloody anger. It was getting expensive throwing crockery so I bought my milk in glass bottles so I could throw them instead.

And so my sessions with Julia continued and she was very, very pleased to hear that I was now expressing anger. A very healthy emotion to be showing as last. I was not hurting so much. My anger was not directed at anyone… well not in the present. Anger is the one emotion that should and usually does come out in short, sharp bursts. Whereas the depressive emotion is the one that lingers and clings and permeates every aspect of waking life. I was glad to feel a lift at last.

Moving and Moving on

After much house searching and almost giving up, I finally found a tiny wooden property in the Yorkshire Dales, in the National Park, within my price range. The property was pretty awful, being a small; static, mobile home but the views and the landscape were stunning. There was a small garden wrapped around the property and there were beautiful views over the open moorland and over to the high fells. It felt like a place for renewal and a place for healing.

It was late autumn when I purchased my little place in the countryside. The property needed quite a bit of work to improve some of the practicalities of such a tiny living space. It measured just 36 feet in length by 10 feet wide - the entire property. Some people have entrance halls bigger than that. But this was all I could afford.

The garden was tidy but looking a little unloved. The garden was one of the main reasons I chose this property; along with the open country views and location. It certainly was not the quality of the property that had anything to do with my decision. As it was Autumn I had to leave the garden in its natural dormant state and wait to see what came up in the Spring. In the meantime my partner and I spend weekends decorating and improving the property over the winter the best we could on limited finances.

I was still working at the Local Authority in the city, which involved commuting an hour each way every day. Some weekends I stayed with my partner, sometimes making it a long weekend so I would not have to do so much commuting as he still lived in the city were my job was. This was also beneficial for Charcoal, my dog, as my partner worked shift-work, so he could spend some time with the dog.

I was relieved to finally find a place of my own with manageable mortgage repayments, and having a garden, which is something I had always wanted. I was looking forward to the spring and to get my hands dirty in the garden.

My health was gradually beginning to improve again now, despite still trying to cope with my awful job and the commuting. I did have many daily symptoms, which I had had for so long that they seemed to be part of everyday life. My energy levels had improved which was a great joy to me. I did have BIG problems with sleeping and many nights I would lie in bed feeling as though I had a furnace burning in the region of my solar plexus. If I put my hand on that area I would feel the heat radiating from my chest. In retrospect, I think this heat was all part of the healing process.

My visits to Julia were beginning to get further apart. This was done partly on Julia's instructions as she wanted me to have sufficient time span between treatments to see how the previous homeopathic remedy took shape and affected my system. Other times Julia would leave it up to me to contact her and arrange for the next visit, when I felt I was ready for it or needed it. Julia was giving me remedies that focused on the endometriosis combined with remedies that worked on my whole constitution and to bolster my immune system.

I still took a selection of supplements, as and when I could afford them. I was still dealing with many residual symptoms regarding sleep and digestive problems. The worst symptom of constant lethargy and tiredness had started to lift from me now, even though I had difficulty sleeping. It was not a sudden thing. It was very gradual, and I hardly noticed the improvement. It was only when I stared to look back that I could gauge that things had moved on quite a bit from where I had been about a year before.

Like I said earlier, I suffered from sleep difficulties. It was difficult to pinpoint what caused it. I tried umpteen things to solve it. I asked Julia about it again and again, but we could not shift it with her help. I tried herbal remedies, alcohol, tiring myself out, and I even had to resort to sleeping tablets from the doctor, as I could not go on any more. I was feeling very jaded and short tempered, and the last thing I needed right now was low energy reserves, as I needed my energy to get better. I had read somewhere that most healing and cell regeneration takes place while we are asleep.

Some of my worst nights were during the full moon, for a period of about 4 nights. On some of these nights I could not sleep at all, even if I had taken a sleeping tablet. Of course sleep is another function of the body that is controlled by a complex and delicate balance of hormones. So it is no surprise that endometriosis sufferers have big problems related to sleep, as it is an illness that is focused around hormonal functions.

I had bouts of constipation and a big problem dealing with Irritable Bowel. It took me a long time to work out all the different foods that were upsetting my system. I also had to sort out when to eat, how much to eat, what I could eat at a given time of day, what to eat with what, which sort of cooking upset me.

My periods were not as bad as they were at the beginning of my endometriosis, but they were not improving as much as I would have liked, considering the amount of time I had been using homeopathy. Julia had forewarned me that many symptoms might get worse before they get better, as this is the nature of healing with homeopathy.

As I mentioned earlier, I was dealing with many layers of healing to address my imbalances which had eventually culminated in my endometriosis. Yes, I called it my endometriosis. I owned up to it eventually. It wasn't 'the endometriosis', a separate thing from me. It was part of me. It was my endometriosis. Nobody else's. I had to deal with it. So I had to listen to it. It - my body, was gradually getting better. It was a slow process and sometimes a painful process. Nobody said healing was going to be easy. But it is a HUGE learning process. Anybody and everybody who has been seriously ill or injured goes through a great learning and humbling experience.

I was no longer living a life like all the friends and people I knew. My life was very different from theirs. My priorities were totally different. My perceptions of my own identity ware totally different. But things were not static. They were changing and I was getting better.

Another Shift

Unfortunately things were not getting any better at work, and nor were they likely to. I still hated it, I hated my jumped up little xxxx of a boss, I hated the building I worked in, and the fact that no one in the organisation cared. Or if they did care they could do nothing about it. Such is the nature of local politics. Obviously I was job hunting in earnest. I applied for loads of jobs, asked around, thought about self-employment, running away, slitting my wrists.

Eventually, finally, at last, I secured another job late in the summer. The post was based much closer to home in a market town on the edge of the National Park. It was a 3-day week with an annual salary just a little under what I was earning at the Local Authority. HORRAY!! I could cope with that nicely. The job was with a brand new voluntary sector project doing community development across a large rural area. I was to be the first officer in post, with total autonomy, able to make my own decisions, set my own time-table and I would be supported by a steering group in the interim until a permanent Management Committee was elected.

I enjoyed the job very much. The flexibility was great and I could work round my health issues. I met some lovely people, travelled round beautiful countryside, and became involved in some very rewarding work.

I was now able to focus more time and energy on my healing and looking after myself. Charcoal and I went for lots and lots of long walks. I was making up for lost time and making the most of the wonderful countryside on my doorstep. I was living in real, vivid, alive countryside. It was hill-farming country with most of the livestock being sheep. There were no crops. No agro-culture with the use of sprays and pesticides. The only crop was the hay crop in the lower meadows and silage for winter feed. The land was fed by muck-spreading - all good natural organic stuff. The weather was in your face, be it summer or winter. There were wild storms, torrential downpours, rainbows, huge sunny skies with swifts and swallows wheeling around the skies. The place was so alive and I loved it. I could really start to feel the energy rising up in me.

My garden was 100% therapy. I was totally hooked. My first summer I was in total bliss. The long evenings were just wonderful and I would still be gardening till the very last bit of light at 10 in the evening. I planted, and repaired, and built things, and spent most of my time outside. It was while I was living here that I experienced the Aurora Borealis. It just makes your jaw drop open. My partner was with me that evening, and we just stared up at it for ages and ages until our necks ached and we were too tired to stay up any longer. Unfortunately I have never seen it since that night.

I did have to pace myself as I was still dealing with endometriosis and its residual symptoms. But only working a 3-day week was exceedingly beneficial to my health and my time. There were times when I felt I wasn't getting anywhere with the healing, but then there would be a sudden realisation of - 'hey, I don't feel so ill, so run down or in so much pain'. The light was coming back into my life.

My social life was beginning to pick up now, but I would be careful not to push myself too far. It was great to be back in the real world now, but it was also great to get back to my little house, away from the noise of the city.

Before I became ill I had started horse riding, and I now felt well enough and strong enough to get back to it. I could not afford it on my income, as horse riding is a very expensive past time. So I thought I would try bartering instead. I put an advert in the local paper offering my services to help out with grooming and mucking out in exchange for some riding. I got a response from a woman living about 5 miles away, and I went riding 2 mornings a week. I had to be up, dressed, breakfasted, drive to her house, and be in the saddle by 8 in the morning. I must have been mad or stupid or both; even on freezing mornings I was there. I could not just turn over in bed and not bother. The horse would be groomed and saddled ready for me, done by the woman's live-in groom, and there was a routine to keep. I learnt so much and become so much more confident with my riding. I feel it also had knock on benefits for my health and for my personal confidence. I always felt exhilarated and alive at the end of each ride.

Slow but Steady

I now had a steady pace in life. I enjoyed my job and it was not taxing me. My little house was not ideal but it was my shelter. I had got to know my neighbours. Friends used to drive up at weekends and come and see me if the weather was good. I loved working in the garden and I had beautiful countryside to go walking in.

My visits to Julia were getting less and less frequent. She was still using a variety of remedies to work on different aspects of healing. I continued with my regime of vitamins and supplements, watched what I ate, and most important I aimed to maintain a positive attitude. My life went on like this with a steady improvement in my health for the next 12 months or so.

I reached a point where I felt so much fitter, most of the acute pain had gone with my periods, I was sleeping better, I could take much longer walks and spend hours working in the garden. My health, my stamina and my outlook had improved so much. I actually started to feel alive, positive, and able to take charge of my life again.

But something was amiss, something was not right. I did not know what it was but I felt as though something in me was stuck. I did not know whether this was physical or metaphysical. But something inside me was blocked, something that could not be shifted with homeopathy. It was a deep and very strong gut knowing. But then I thought I was being absolutely stupid and the feeling would pass and I would carry on as usual.

Then again, I had the same feeling once more. A strong sense something was not right. I could not fathom it out. I felt strong, I felt fit and healthier than I had done in years. I was in the fresh air a lot of the time, walking, and horse riding, careful with my diet. I do not actually feel ill at all. So why do I get this .... feeling.

This went on for about 2 months, and I felt as fit as a fiddle but had this little niggling voice inside my head ...... there is something wrong, something is not right. It was that little voice, my intuition. I had to listen to it as it was getting louder and louder.

My gut feeling was that I needed another look inside to check what was going on. I needed another laparoscopy. Why did I want to put myself through another operation when I felt so much better, I had no symptoms of any sort, but I just knew it had to be done?

I talked about this to a few people and most of them said I should listen to my gut feeling. I made an appointment to see Julia and I discussed with her all that had been going on. She immediately said, if that is how I feel, and the feeling is so strong, and then I should definitely act on it. She was adamant about this.

I then went to see my doctor. Fortunately, I had a forward thinking doctor who was totally happy with me to follow the self-help route with my healing, and supported me if I needed it. I told him of all my progress to date, about my intuitive feelings of a need for another operation despite there being no symptoms, and what Julia had said. My doctor respected my approach to the whole situation and was willing to refer me to a gynaecologist again.

As I was living in a different area from when I was first diagnosed with endometriosis, I knew I would be going to the local hospital which was much more modern, had better facilities and more up to date equipment. A total contrast to my first hospital experience.

My doctor informed me that there was a new gynaecologist at the hospital, with up to date training, along with new, state of the art laser surgery equipment. I knew laser surgery was much less invasive than conventional surgery should I need any surgical procedure doing.

With the information that had been given to me regarding the new resources at the local hospital, along with the advice I had received, I felt that things had conspired for me to pursue the avenue of having another operation. I was confident and secure in myself and knew I was doing absolutely the right thing. Like I said earlier, I had absolutely no worrying symptoms, no pain, and I felt very fit and energetic. The only symptoms I did have were the residual symptoms of an immune system that had taken a good knock. I had the occasional night where sleep was still a problem and I still had to be careful to watch what I ate with regards to Irritable Bowel.

So I proceeded with my request for another Laparoscopy, and an appointment was made for me to go and see the new gynaecologist at the hospital to discuss the possibility of investigative surgery. It needs to be noted here that this story is based in the UK, where health treatment is free through the National Health Service. For me to convince the gynaecologist to perform a Laparoscopy, I would need to be pretty convincing that something was wrong under normal circumstances. But I had no symptoms; how was my request to be received!

It was now mid summer and I went to my appointment with all sorts of mixed feelings and emotions, and a swirl of thoughts going through my head. But despite all those thoughts and emotions, I still felt a deep confident calm inside me. It turned out that the gynaecologist was originally from Sri Lanka which boded well, as he was very sympathetic to my self-help approach for my healing. I told him my entire story.

He paused for a while; he looked in his diary and asked me when I would like to come in for my operation. I was wonderfully surprised. I was anticipating a good dose of cynicism from the gynaecologist at least. My greatest fear was that the gynaecologist would tell me to stop wasting hospital and doctor time when I had no symptoms. But I think the positive conspiracy deepened, as he was a 'tuned in' younger doctor, who was willing to listen to me. I mean he really listened. I also think his cultural background helped. Yes he was trained in the West, but his cultural background originated in the East where healing and medicine has a much more holistic approach.

As I was given the option to choose a date for my operation, which was almost unheard of in the UK health service, I decided to take advantage of this. I did not want to be held up in bed recovering from an operation in the middle of the summer so I asked if I could go into hospital at the end of the summer when I would not miss the garden so much, and the weather would not be so glorious. And so it was booked.

My big problem now was what to do about my job. I was the only person working on the project. There was no admin support worker, or any other form of back-up staff. I ran the entire project by myself. I did not know what would happen or what would be found during my operation. I did not know how long I would need to recover. And I could not very easily shut down the project for an unspecified length of time with ongoing work in progress.

I thought long and hard about this and the only solution I could come up with was to resign from the project. It was a very tricky situation to be in. Had I been in a job where other staff could stand in for me, and then there would be no problem. So I resolved to stop work and hope the future would bring new opportunities. In the next meeting of the Steering Group of the project I discussed with the members what I was dealing with and what my decision was. My news was received with respect and support. It was decided to advertise for a replacement for me straight away, and the new person would come into the post with 2 weeks overlap before I left so that skills and advice could be passed on.

Decisive Discovery

It was now September, I had finished my job and I went into hospital for my second Laparoscopy. It had been nearly five years since my first operation and my diagnosis. I had not touched any conventional drug treatment. I had used only Homeopathy, supplements, diet management and lots of positive thinking. I was fit and felt healthy and now going onto the operating table again purely because I had an intuitive message that simply would not go away.

I had my operation mid morning. I came round from the anaesthetic and found I was back on the ward. Once again I felt awful from the effects of the operation and I felt very tender and sore. The worst feeling was this sensation as though a sword had been run through my rib cage. What the hell was it. The nurse told me it was the effects of the gas used in the operation, which had been pumped into my abdomen so that my internal organs moved out of the way and the surgeon could see easier during the operation. I was told that the gynaecologist would be round the next day to tell me how it went.

I did not come round properly from the anaesthetic for hours but every time I tried to move this pain in my rib cage kept shifting around and was causing me agony. (I don't remember suffering this same pain when I had my first laparoscopy.) I laid there in a daze just thinking and wondering what had been found during my operation. I spent the night drifting in and out of sleep.

The next morning the pains in my rib cage continued to shift and dart around, causing awful sensations. I had to keep changing position to try and escape this pain. The nurse on duty said I would be ready to go home that day after I had seen the gynaecologist. I did want to see the gynaecologist, desperately, but I did not want to go home. There would be no one at home to look after me, so I asked the nurse if she could enquire if I could stay one more night. She said she would make enquiries and let me know.

I waited and waited, I dozed off. Woke up again. I could not stand the suspense. Then finally my gynaecologist arrived on the ward doings his rounds. He came up to my bedside and smiled.

He immediately informed me that I had no active endometriosis. It had all dried up. He said he had done a good search around my insides. What he did find was a small to medium size cyst on my right ovary which he had treated, and that he had also freed any adhesions in my abdomen that had been left behind.

No active Endometriosis ………….. that was all I could hear, those were the only words I could focus on **NO ACTIVE ENDOMETRIOSIS**.

Then gradually I realised what my intuition had been telling me about was the cyst and the old adhesions. My inner voice was telling me something was 'stuck', something needed to be cleared out. If I had not listened to my inner voice that cyst could have got bigger if left un-checked. I had listened to my body and my intuition, and I was proved right to pay attention. That inner voice had been constant and persistent over a period of months.

I went home after my operation with so many feelings - joy, amazement, curiosity, and relief. I rested up for a week or so after my operation. I then contacted Julia, my homeopath to tell her the news. She was obviously delighted and pleased for me.

The reason for my second laparoscopy was based purely on a very strong intuitive feeling of the need to be checked internally. I felt something was amiss but I had no idea what, and I had no symptoms. In fact I was fitter than I had been in many years.

My homeopath felt that this last cyst was the last physical evidence, the final manifestation of the disease. It was as though all the toxic debris and residue of endometriosis had been moped up into one place, ready for the final treatment.

My intuition to get checked internally despite feeling really fit and well was immensely strong and would not go away. I tried to ignore it, knowing how fit I felt, but in the end my intuition was screaming at me. I had worked with my homeopath for 4 years and together we went through 'layers' of healing, finally getting to the root causes of my ill health and endometriosis.

The disease was finally laid to rest with the support of homeopathic remedies and the many steps I took to help myself. The final cyst on my ovary was the last 'process' in my healing, strange as that may sound. This cyst made my intuition kick in, which enabled me to get this last physical evidence cleared up once and for all.

The timing of events in this story still fascinates me today. Just at the time I felt I was ready and needed to have another operation, the new gynaecologist had just arrived with the relevant training and the new laser equipment. It is peculiar how the universe sometimes conspires for events to synchronise in time.

Continuing my Healing

Of course the story does not finish there. Having the last operation was not the final 'magic wand' and life is happy ever after. I knew the real risk of endometriosis returning if I was not careful with my health. I also knew that stress plays a major part in 90% of all known illnesses and I did not want to take any risks.

I was now out of work, and in hindsight I should have finished work long before I did, but life's events and circumstances meant that I could not. I needed a secure job to secure a mortgage, to have a secure roof over my head and so on. I had already lost one home to the property developers - never again.

I was now out of work, recovering from an operation, borrowing money to pay my mortgage in the short term, and wondering how the hell do I cope. My partner was very supportive and helped me out the best he could. I was now claiming sickness benefit from the State, but was getting no help with my housing costs and I had to borrow the money to pay my mortgage. I would get State help with my mortgage payments after 6 months of being on welfare benefit, but that seemed light-years away.

I started to learn to live on my wits. I knew how to feed myself well, and reasonably cheaply. Over the years I had bought many of my clothes from charity shops, so I would continue to do the same. I took on some sewing jobs for a friend of mine to earn some 'pin money' - literally. But I knew money was going to be very, very tight. There was not much I could do about it in the immediate future. I had to recover from the operation and I had to look after my health.

As soon as I was fit enough I went back to horse riding, taking it gently at first. I originally started riding around the time I finished college and I loved it immediately. Mind you, my first ride ever was straight out to open countryside; it was a white-knuckle ride, but I got back to the riding yard exhilarated and had caught the bug. There is no way you can be depressed while horse riding, and it is a great way to take your mind off things. You are so busy concentrating on what you are doing at that moment in time. It is one of those activities that make you be right 'in the moment'. It is excellent exercise and I also feel it is a great method of massaging the internal organs to keep them supple and to keep the blood flowing.

I then reached a point where I wanted to get back to my artwork and do something creative. I had more time on my hands now and it had been a long time since I had done anything creative. I did not know where to start or what I wanted to do. I had always enjoyed working with textiles. The variety of materials is almost limitless ranging from silk to sacking. Then I picked up a prospectus of evening classes at the local college. They were running an accredited course in Creative Textiles, so I registered. The course was great and the techniques and skills I learnt were brilliant.

I managed like this for a few months but my money was getting tighter and tighter. I was beginning to get stressed by my financial situation. I was still able to obtain sickness benefit from the state, but it was a pittance. I had to get more money from somewhere. I decided the only thing I could do was to earn some money through the 'black economy'. I looked for a couple of cleaning jobs in my area. It transpired that the woman I went horse riding with was looking for a cleaner so I started working for her 2 mornings a week. This helped to ease the cash flow.

And so I managed to limp along financial like this for a while. I had to come off the sickness benefit and went on to unemployment benefit. I still had to work on the black economy, and was conscious that I could get caught and prosecuted for doing this work. It was a worrying time. But the prospect of finding another good job with the problems of the economic climate, as well as living in a rural area, was rather remote. I had started to check out the job situation, but things did not look promising.

My little property was beginning to show the ravages of age despite the work we had put into it. Over the winter, after my operation, the rain had got into the roof and it was now sagging badly. My partner had to cut a length of strong timber and put a support in the middle of the roof span on the inside of the property. This was serious. We sat down and discussed what I could do. The place needed a new roof and I needed some money. My partner said he could replace the roof with a much nicer apex roof to replace the flat roof it had. Most of the work involved working with timber which he was happy to do. After looking at my limited options, I obtained the money to repair the roof by cashing in the value of my endowment policy on my mortgage, which had just enough value to pay for the materials.

This was another very stressful time. The building work seemed to take ages but it could not go any faster. Every time the weather was bad the work had to stop. And there were only the weekends that it could be done.

I was beginning to feel very ill at ease about living in this situation. I had only managed to obtain a mortgage on this property by technically re-mortgaging my partner's property which he had paid cash for. The actual mortgage policy was in my name. And here I was living and paying for a property that was loosing value, not gaining it, like bricks and mortar would. The property was now starting to require lots of work. The reality was that the property should have been demolished and a brand new mobile home put on the site. The property complex where I lived was on the edge of a small village and it consisted of 10 of these mobile homes. Some of them had been replaced with brand new units which were very luxurious and much bigger than mine.

It was beginning to feel that my time here at my little wooden house in the countryside was coming to an end. There was too much stress. Too many problems to resolve. I could not afford a new unit to replace the one I had bought. My chances of finding work again in a rural area were very slim. I was beginning to suffer from social deprivation. I had also received notice from County Court for non-payment of Poll Tax from the previous financial year. I had not paid it because I could not afford it.

This despicable tax was part of Margaret Thatchers' legacy to the general populace of the UK. It was a tax payable by every single person over the age of 18 (I think) no matter what your income, your circumstances, your assets; every one had to pay. There were pensioners going into prison because they refused to pay it, as they could not afford it. Hundreds of thousands of people were getting into trouble because of this tax. People who had obeyed the law all their lives were now getting criminal records. And so the same happened to me.

One wet miserable afternoon, bailiffs from the Local Authority turned up on my doorstep wanting to know how I was going to pay my unpaid tax. They said they could not leave the property until I had come to some agreement. All I could do was inform them to take me to court. I was on welfare benefit, I was unfit to work, I had no savings, and there was nowhere I could borrow money from. One guy rang back to his main office relaying my situation. He fed back to his colleague at the other end of the phone that there were no valuable assets on the property to take in lieu of payment. And so I had to sign a document saying I could not pay and court proceedings would be processed.

Fortunately I was able to submit a guilty plea by post without the humility of going to court. I included all my financial details and circumstances and posted off my plea. I was asked to repay the unpaid tax, which was about £300, at £5 per week. Even this was too much on my budget. After discussing this with friends, one particularly astute friend of mine told me that as long as I paid something, anything, then I cannot be taken to court for non-payment, as I would be paying something. For the next 9 months I went to the small local government office in the next village to pay a token gesture each and every week. Sometimes it was as little as £2. I did not care about the inconvenience it caused the beaurocrats; my life had been totally inconvenienced too and a lot of stress had been caused.

I decided it was time to try and sell the place for whatever I could get, but I definitely had to cover the cost of paying back the mortgage. My partner and I decided that the best plan of action was to finish the roof and then decorate the interior to a suitable standard so as to attract a sale.

It was spring when the roof was finished and it looked great. It totally changed the appearance of the property as well as the feel of it. On the interior we decided to leave the ceiling vaulted into the apex and not to fill it in with a flat ceiling. It looked great from the outside. The inside was a totally different story. There were entire wall panels missing, heavy duty electric cables hanging loose everywhere, light fittings to refit, doors to re-hang, it was a mess. But we were doing the best we could to get it back into shape again.

Then one day there was a knock on the door. It was a Sunday afternoon. A couple in their 60's stood there and they introduced themselves. They said that they understood that I was going to put my place on the market in the future when the work had been done. My neighbours who were friends of theirs had informed them of this, and would I mind if they came in and had a look.

I was totally surprise. I apologised for the mess but they said they understood completely. They explained that they would like to retire to the area as they loved it so much and it would be great to have their friends as neighbours as they used to live close together before. The husband explained he was a retired architect and would I mind if he came back in the week to do some measuring. I said it was no problem and we made arrangements. I did not make too much of their visit considering the state of the property.

The husband came back as arranged, did some measuring and said he and his wife could be very interested in buying the place in its present condition. He took my phone number, said he would ring in a few days after they had done their sums and off they went to see their friends up the road.

I was now beginning to hold my breath. This would be the absolute ideal situation. I would not have to finish the renovation work, I would not have to find the money to do the final renovation work, I would not have to pay to advertise and sell the house through an agent, I could pay off the mortgage, they were not short of money, I could ask a reasonable price without selling up in a financial panic; they were obviously very interested in the location, so I had the trump card here.

Sure enough, the husband rang me 3 days later, said they were very interested and made me an offer. I said I wanted to think about the offer, and said I would ring him back. I did not want to seem too keen and bite his hand off. I had already set my own price that I had planned to ask when selling, to cover repaying the mortgage plus a bit extra, as I knew the value of the land would have increased, if not that of the property. His offer had been a bit low so I wanted to bargain. I rang him back and told him my final figure was between his original offer and my original price. He agreed there and then on the phone and I had a sale.

Things moved very fast after that. They wanted the purchase to go through quickly so that they had the summer to demolish the old unit and put a brand new one on site. I had 4 weeks in which to pack the remainder of my stuff up, tie up any loose ends and move out.

More Moving

It was a huge wrench moving away from my lovely garden and the stunning countryside. But things do not stay the same in life; we cannot remain static. I knew my time there had come to a natural conclusion. Everything had happened so quickly. I had no time to plan or organise anything and so I moved in with my partner on a temporary basis.

The timing of the sale coincided with other events in my life. I had been doing a lot of artwork and had organised a solo exhibition at a small gallery in the city. The date of this was 2 weeks after the completion date for the sale of the house. Things were manic and I was rushing round like a headless chicken. The exhibition went well and I sold a few small items of work which gave my ego a little boost. Lots of my friends came to the private viewing evening and I felt as though I had got back to a place of normal living again.

Then about 2 weeks after the exhibition I decided I had better take Charcoal to the vets as she had been limping badly on and off for a few weeks. They could not find anything obvious and asked for her to stay overnight and have some x-rays in the morning. I went down to the vets the following evening anticipating to be told of a simple sprain or something.

Charcoal had bone cancer. Just writing that last sentence has brought up a huge wave of grief. It is years since she has been gone but I still miss her. She was with me through thick and thin. Through all the pain and agony I went through with my endometriosis. Through all the agonies and distress I went through with life. We did have lots of good times together and I took her everywhere with me. She was so laid back. She never needed to be put on a lead, her road sense was brilliant. She was very sociable and everybody who met her just adored her. There were quite a few of my friends who were in tears when they heard that I had decided to have her put to sleep. She was obviously in pain, which is why she was limping. There was no treatment for it and the vet said she was probable in pain even when she was at rest. I could not sit by and let her suffer like that just to appease my own needs. I cried for weeks after the event. One of the saddest events of my life.

There had been huge shifts happening in my life and all happening so quickly. Selling my home and resolving all the anxiety around property maintenance and money, having my first solo exhibition and the death of my canine companion. I was dealing with relief, grief, fear, fulfilment, and a whole mixed bag of emotions.

I just went into free-fall for the next couple of months. I had to recover from tiredness, the stress of moving, the stress of the input into my exhibition, and the grief I was feeling. It was time to rest a while.

Making up for Lost Time

I will briefly summarise my story beyond the initial healing stage of my body. Yes I had conquered my battle against endometriosis. The man in the hospital told me, my body had told me. I now needed to heal my soul. I also needed to make up for lost time, lost experiences, lost opportunities. I also needed to be sure that I could continue my life in good health.

I did still have residual symptoms and I would have occasional setbacks. Just as the body can be left with a limp after a bad accident or left with a scar after damaged tissue. Having an illness leaves a residue in the body. The cells have memory and sometimes old symptoms can return for a while just to remind you to be careful how you treat your body. I too had been damaged. I had been damaged physically and mentally. This was now a time for me to assimilate what I had been through and to think about where I needed to go now in my life.

My temporary move to my partners place turned out to be a bit longer than anticipated and I was there for about a year. I did not have any concrete plans of my own; I just wanted to ease up on life. I did not even want to take on the responsibility of running my own home which is why I did not look for rented accommodation.

I found another contact where I was able to barter for my horse riding. I could write a book on all the adventures, the people, the animals and the events that took place on this smallholding. I would be there with sandwiches and a flask of coffee at least 4 half days a week. I witnessed foals being born, goats being born, and there was one particular horse that gave me the confidence to go out riding on my own. He was an older, confident horse who could look after himself, and he had lots of character. I loved him to bits.

I wanted to get involved in new activities now and new interests. I was ready to spread my wings. I went to a music event one evening and I was watching a mixed group of people of all ages playing a load of drums and percussion instruments, playing some brilliant Samba rhythms. It was great; it was energetic; I thought I could do that. I made enquiries with one of the members after they had finished, and found out that they were an open access Samba School and I was welcome to go to their rehearsals and join. Even better, they were based in the city where I was living. So I went down on the designated evening, had some instruments shoved my way and jumped in at the deep end. About 3 weeks later I was joining these people on stage at my first gig. It was a huge buzz and I loved it. Music had come into my life.

I ended up playing gigs with these people all over the place including Nottinghill Carnival, and joined 250 other Sambistas in an event in Belfast, taking part in the first non-sectarian march to take place in Belfast for about 50 years. I met some wonderful people and my social life really took off.

I also started doing African drumming at this time. This too had spin offs with new friends, playing at concerts and festivals and having lots of fun, as well as bringing new variety to my social life.

My relationship with my partner was beginning to break down. We both wanted different things in life now. We did both try to compromise but it was not working. Eventually we parted and I moved into a spare room at a friend's house. I still had no job and I felt I would have great difficulty in getting my career back on track. I had applied for a number of interesting jobs, but the matter of my illness and being out of work kept being referred to at interviews. This happened again and again. I was beginning to get loud warning bells.

I started to lie on my job applications and not mention the fact I had been ill and been out of work. This made obtaining references very tricky sometimes. I was getting nowhere in my job hunt, and in the end I gave up. The job market was as tough as ever, and for a woman with a gap on her CV and a history of a serious illness, and then the prospect of securing a job was very slim.

I gave up looking for work; it was a fruitless waste of time. I went back to looking for bits of work on the black economy again to keep myself financially afloat. I had a small amount of savings now from the sale of the property, but I was not going to touch that for cost of living expenses. I did spend some of it soon after the sale and purchased a small second-hand camper van. My partner and I went off for long weekends in it while we were still together and I loved it. The total freedom, with much more luxury than camping under canvas.

Around this time I started weight training to increase my strength and stamina. I also did training in healing and then went on to do Aromatherapy/Massage training. I was like a sponge. I had a lot of catching up to do. I was starting to live again.

By now I had a clean slate, no determined path and no responsibilities. I had no job, no partner, no permanent home of my own, not even any pets. The possibilities and options open to me were limitless. Instead of standing on the edge of the abyss like I had in the past, I now stood on the horizon with a 360-degree panorama of possibilities.

Spreading my Wings

I spent just over a year living in the city in lodgings with my friend and her family, with life happily bumbling along, getting involved more and more with the music and drumming, socialising more, getting fitter and stronger at the gym and doing horse riding. My life was now about living rather than surviving. I had weekends away, went to residential music festivals, went to France in the campervan with a friend of mine, and lots of other normal every day things that so many people take for granted. I was getting back on an even keel.

After this recuperation period I started to take stock of my life and think of things I wanted to do with my life. In an ideal world I would have liked to recover my career, but the omens were not looking good to achieve this. Granted, I could have downgraded my aspirations and obtained work in a factory or doing menial office work. But I knew in my heart that this move would have added insult to injury; after all I had gone through; to find myself in a dead-end job, which would not improve my CV or my prospects of obtaining rewarding work.

After much soul searching, talking to friends, and researching different options, I decided to go travelling. I wanted to have some adventures now. I wanted to achieve things which were denied me in the past. I had to be rather creative in my planning, as my funds were limited. So I decided to travel round the UK doing voluntary work. I found an organisation which administered the placement of volunteers on organic farms and smallholdings around the country, and I set up a series of placements.

Having put my few belongings into storage in the cellar of my friend's house, I loaded the car with basic camping equipment, a few decent clothes and some working gear, and set off to work round the UK for the summer. It was hard work, I met some interesting people, I learnt a lot, sweated a lot, got dirty a lot, explored all the local areas, and I had the freedom to move on to my next placement whenever I felt like it.

At the end of the summer I returned to base and then started planning a winter trip to the Far

East, with the aim of backpacking for 4 months. I set off in the November, travelled round Malaysia, Thailand, and parts of Indonesia, and returned in early March. It was a trip with mixed experiences, some good, some bad, but on the whole it was a nourishing and fulfilling journey.

On my return I decided to make the move to another part of the UK, to discover a new area, but also be closer to my family. I had already decided on my new location after talking to different people I met on my travels. I went in search of accommodation in the area and to secure a job, any job, so that I could finance the move. I did not know anyone in the area, and all my friends said I was very brave to move on my own. I told them that if it did not work out and I was not happy, then I could simply pack up my belongings and move back.

Well it did work out. It all worked out wonderfully. After settling in, making new friends, getting a better job, I met a wonderful man. There was chemistry between us as soon as we met, and it was only a matter of months before I moved in with him. I was absolutely sure and confident that this was the man I wanted to be with….. and the rest is history as they say.

Conclusion to my Story

This has been a long and winding story but I felt the whole picture needed to be coloured in. As I said earlier, we are the sum total of all our experiences. I took the bull by the horns all those years ago. I dealt with many demons and many harrowing experiences. This story does not include the details of other significant things that happened to me. Like the operation to have a breast lump removed, the scare relating to my father's health; trying to bond with my mother on holiday, having not seen her for over 20 years, and finding the roles reversed.

I have come through a lot and I wanted to put my journey through illness and back to health into context for my readers so they get to understand the whole picture; get to understand my mind set, where I stood socially, economically, practically, as all these circumstances have an influence on your health and well-being.

There were many people who supported me through this. At the same time there were also people who disappeared into the woodwork, never to be seen again. The people who helped me saw me at my worst, and then they watched me grow and develop and become what I am today.

Throughout the problems in my life, the distress and torment caused by endometriosis, I never totally doubted that I would get rid of this illness. On the surface I did wander from my faith at times. I did sometimes think and feel I was chasing a false hope. But somewhere deep inside me I had a strange and strong sense of knowing that this was not going to last forever, that I was going to be rid of it and that I would move on in life.

I kept telling myself over and over and over again - THIS IS GOING TO GO AWAY, I AM NOT GOING TO TOLERATE IT, THIS IS NOT WHAT MY LIFE IS SUPPOSED TO BE ABOUT, THIS IS NOT MY DESTINY.

I had a destiny somewhere else. I had a destiny which included the positive things in life, the colours of life, my creativity, my sense of adventure, and my sense of fulfilment. A life that involved freedom of movement, freedom of choice, freedom to fly.

Another Success Story of Healing from Endometriosis

A few years ago, the first edition of this book was purchased by a woman in Morocco. I did not get any immediate feedback from her. Then suddenly out of the blue I received an email communication from Ingrid, saying how fit and well she was, having taken on board the advice and supportive ideas from my book. She said she would send me her full story when she had more time on her hands.

Here is Ingrid's Endo Healing story....

Part One

'I had endometriosis for a couple of years and in 2001 I had to go to France for an operation. The surgeon, who was very skilful, took away the endo-cysts and one ovary and said there is no other cure than surgical removal. He added half jokingly, while smoking one cigarette after the other, that that was a fortunate thing, since if there was a cure; he would be out of work... Incredible, isn't it? Allopathic (traditional) doctors don't learn in their medical schools that there is always a cause behind each disease and that the body is always doing its best to heal, and that the body is programmed in a "win win" mode.

Then my sister, who also had suffered from the same disease, told me to think about what the illness represents symbolically. It took me several years to grasp that question, let alone, finding the answer. But it indeed helped me to have a more spiritual and holistic attitude and to search for answers inside myself.

Anyway, 2 years after the surgery, I got the endo back again, and my female gyno told me that hysterectomy was the only solution. She added to state that the uterus is only a muscle anyway, and that I didn't need it anymore, and that I should go home and start doing the grief-work of my uterus and come back after the summer vacation to take everything out.

I was 44 years old; I was horrified, but very glad that I did not take her words for granted. I went to 5 different doctors and they all agreed on the same solution: surgery. But I refused. I went online and started my personal research by consulting the website: www.curezone.com and it was there that I found Carolyn's site www.endo-resolved.com. I immediately purchased and downloaded her book (Reclaim Your Life- Your Guide to Healing of Endometriosis) in PDF format and read it from cover to cover. What a relief to read her healing story!

Then I went to 2 holistic naturopaths. One in Marrakech and one in Casablanca, - each were completing one another. From the first one I got a deep-acting homeopathic treatment and she also put me on a STRICT diet. She said that she has helped many people with many different health-problems but only the ones who followed the diet for at least 3 months were cured. I said, "Sure, I'm enough motivated."

I had been eating what you would call a more or less healthy diet, with a lot of vegetables, but I had had a tendency to eat between meals and to indulge in chocolate, sweets and ice cream. From now on, however, no more sugary snacks.

This was the diet which could be called a cleansing diet:

No sugar, no diary products, no white rice, no coffee or black tea, no meat, fish only from time to time, and no GLUTEN (no bread), no eggs, no warm pressed oils, no hydrogenated fats (found in nearly all biscuits, candy, Mars bars etc and peanut butter.)

Replace white rice with brown rice, replace white sugar items, if desperate, with soaked almonds, or make a fruit cake with gluten free flour and dates, figs, sweetened with a tiny sprinkle of the natural plant Stevia (I imported it from the USA).

Replace the protein from the excluded meat with proteins from vegetables like Avocado, lentils, pulses in general, a well as SPROUTED GRAINS: Sprouted mung beans, lentils, Alfa Alfa, etc. Replace the industrially warm pressed oils with cold pressed virgin oil. Replace BREAD with gluten free bread or rice biscuits. You can get all advice you need from your Naturopath and from your local Health Store. (There is also advice on the diet for endometriosis here at Endo Resolved)

No more unhealthy snacks! It took a while for me to adapt to this diet, and the most difficult time was when I was invited and during Christmas and other holidays visiting family, who always want to prepare huge rich meals and sugary ice cream for desert. Every time I had to remind myself of what all the doctors had told me, reread parts of Carolyn's book in order to re-motivate myself.

Part Two

The DIET was:

BREAKFAST: in winter: corn flour porridge or millet porridge spiced with cinnamon and cardamom and raisins) delicious) with or without soaked prunes, figs and apricots. In summer fruit, and freshly made carrot/ cucumber/beetroot juice. Very cleansing and invigorating. A lot of alkaline mineral water, and at 11 o'clock a snack if necessary. Soaked almonds and nuts, dried fruit, figs, dates or an apple, pear.

LUNCH: 70 - 80 % raw food not to forget the sprouts and some boiled potatoes, brown rice or beans or vegetables. Dressing without vinegar since its acid, replace vinegar with lemon juice.

DINNER: Steamed or cooked vegetables for dinner Talk to your Naturopath about how to get all the necessary proteins. In America there are many specialists on that subject, many many more than where I live, here in Morocco, where everybody, without exception, eats meat twice a day.

I also got different essential oils to put on the liver, or swallow a few drops. One was for cleansing the liver, one was to help digestion...I had slow metabolism and VERY slow digestion. I had to learn how to EAT SLOWLY, which still today is a big problem. I have a tendency to just throw in the food in my mouth and swallow....

At some point I put CASTOR oil on my pelvis area as described in Carolyn's book. It was a bit complicated and messy, but since I knew it was a very old and well-documented prescription, I persevered. I also got the prescription to take Omega 3 oil, either from fish of from linseed. I also took Evening Primrose oil.

A Russian friend here in Casablanca gave me a Russian cure that I could prepare myself. My friend had used it to clear out a "fibrome" and I found that it could not be harmful so I might as well try it. You break up walnuts and gather the lining which separates the two departments. You put them in a jar and pour vodka or, as in my case, cognac on it. Then you store it for 2 weeks, before you start taking 15 drops three times a day for three months. I have no idea of what the active ingredient can be in this TINTCURE but maybe it contributed?

The second Naturopath gave me cleansing herbs to boil and to drink as herb-tea. It tasted horrible, but my motivation was strong enough to endure. The second Naturopath also checked my Ph level and noticed that my body fluids were acid. The diet slowly corrected this imbalance. Lately, I have read a book by Dr Robert Young, called The PH-MIRACLE which describes and explains the utter importance of having the body fluids at the right pH level - alkaline. You can visit his website www.thephmiracle.com and learn more.

I gather that all the bean sprouts that I grew in my kitchen helped me a lot to get enough live enzymes and alkalizing food. I also bumped into the natural anti inflammatory – SERRAPEPTASE (This is one of the enzymes found in Vitalzym which has been mentioned here on the website at Endo Resolved) which is the laboratory cultivation of an enzyme from the silkworm, known to "consume" dead tissue, since the silkworm needs to digest the very coarse leaves from the Mulberry tree. The official name of this drug went under DAZEN and I think that's for French speaking countries.

I chose to have 2 Naturopaths, especially as the first one lived in Marrakech, which is three hours from here. I needed to go and see someone once a week, and later twice a month to be able to persevere and stay motivated.

I also looked into the emotional issues behind contacting this disease. I saw a NLP coach who was very intuitive and together we cleared out many deep issues about inherited femininity and Motherhood from my Mother and my Grandmother.

You might think that you need a very huge budget to do all these things to have several Naturopaths and NLP coaches. But no, it doesn't need to get that expensive and if you really, really desire something deeply and that you take one step in that direction, the universe will help you with the second step. I got this counselling over at least 2 years and it was indeed worth every penny!!!

The very best investment for me was counselling in holistic Naturopathy and Cognitive or NLP therapy. Rebirthing therapy is also something that I practice at least twice a yea, since here in Casablanca we have an association that organizes seminars for Rebirthing with rebirthers from abroad. This is a kind of breath therapy that can be very helpful, and indeed powerful. It was founded by the American Leonard Orr and Sondra Ray.

Part Three

Apart from Carolyn's book, that got me started from the beginning and without which I would never have even TRIED to give my body a second chance with naturopathy...(Thank you Carolyn, I'm deeply grateful that you wrote the book and put it out online so we all get access to it.) Apart from that first book the books that helped me were:

All books by DEEPAK CHOPRA. Wow, he articulates so many complex things about the body mind connection in such beautiful and simple ways; he is my absolute favourite author. If I lived in America I would definitely try to go to one of his lectures.

Louise Hay: also an American bestseller. All her books are very helpful. Check out Hay House online. She cured herself from cancer, a much more severe illness than Endometriosis. She has different cassettes treating different SELF HELP subjects that I listen to in the car. It helps me to be more positive and she is an excellent role model.

Barbara Wren: a British teacher and researcher in Natural Nutrition, head of the College of Natural Nutrition in London and in Essex. She healed herself from Multiple Sclerosis, and then gave birth to a fifth child. I managed to get a copy of one of her lectures and I listen to this over and over to understand more about the subtle ways of the body. If you send me your post addresses, I will be more than happy to send you a copy of this cassette about healing the body.

Now we come to YOGA. Before I started to take responsibility for my own healing and evolution I TALKED a lot about Yoga and how cool it was without even practicing it...Lazy character I suppose...

Then a good friend pulled me into it. Ashtanga Yoga. Now I understand and feel from the inside what miracles it works especially when you have lack of energy in the pelvis area and lack of consciousness down there!

I also found on the American website: www.yogajournal.com a chapter on which poses are best to ease different ailments etc. I put in endometriosis in their little search engine and found a whole chapter on Yoga and Endo Excellent! After 2 years HARD STRUGGLE to get into the practice, I have now finally worked myself up to a level where I long for doing my practice. It works like an injection. It opens up the hips and builds up strength. I can NOT do it straight after getting up in the morning, but feel more ready and LESS STIFF after about 15 min after I have had the chance to wake up a bit and loosen up. It energises the whole pelvis area and helped clean it out of mucus and blood. I now practice a few specific postures everyday that worked for me.

Then after 2 years I got a terrible pain in my left breast and feared the worst, went to see the gyno just for that, and had actually stopped fearing that the gyno would cut out my womb. I felt more secure in my body, even though the breast pain was scary. So I entered the docs practice with the printout of Carolyn's book in my hands! Not a very diplomatic way of addressing the doc I realized afterwards. The doc felt entirely threatened, and no wonder! How come somebody DARES question their authority? !

The doc said, after having looked at the x-ray of the breast that all was OK, and anyway if you happen to contract breast cancer, it doesn't hurt. So my pain was hormonal. Then she did an ecography ultrasound scan of my uterus. She shook her head and mumbled something about mucus...then the examination was over and we didn't even talk about the endometriosis catastrophe since 2 years and the planned for hysterectomy. She was unpleasant and stressed, and dismissed me quickly out of her office. Not until I got home I read the conclusion of the ultrasound which stated in a very undecipherable handwriting - no cysts, no sign of endometriosis.

I was SO HAPPY and could hardly believe her words. I was also angry at her lack of civic responsibility of surpassing her docs ego and telling me that I no longer had endometriosis and didn't need hysterectomy anymore! She didn't even tell me!

To conclude and re-enforce her observation, I went to another totally new gyno who didn't know anything about my history. I asked him several times, is everything clear? No cysts? And he said everything looked absolutely clear and OK. The uterus had some mucus but not anything alarming. Then, when I had got this second opinion and statement I told him that 5 gynos had planned Hysterectomy for me. I told him how I had gone into natural healing and started yoga. To my surprise, this was a positive and open gyno, who even took the business card of my yoga teacher.

I have noticed that when I fail to eat healthily and gulp a lot of bread and sugar, I get pain in the pelvis again. It's a reminder that my body is a bit fragile to certain elements. So I go on a diet again. No bread, no sugar. A lot of bean sprouts. And then after a couple of weeks of that diet I feel no pain again.

End of Part Three

Wow, now I have to rest a bit, I am home with flu, it gave me enough time to write this, but now I must rest again. Talk to you later ladies. AND don't despair, there are several solutions out there for your symptoms and ailments and diseases! Trust and pray and ask for guidance

and it will come to you. It was a pleasure sharing this. Hope you can take benefit from my story.'

Love Ingrid in Casablanca, Morocco. April 2007

Part Two

An Overview of Endometriosis

Endometriosis

This section deals with the main known facts of endometriosis, covering an over-view of what endometriosis is, the symptoms, diagnosis, treatment, cause and finally, how this disease affects the different areas of your life. You may feel the need to skip this part of the book if you have already read a lot of the basic facts about endometriosis, but I have included it here to provide a reference for those of you who require this information.

You may however find the information in part three to be somewhat disturbing, which covers some revealing and sometimes serious facts I found during my research. Some of you may have read about these issues before, i.e. toxins in the environment, toxic toiletries, and the economics of health care; but here I have gone into more depth than you may have read before, with the aim of linking subjects together, rather than leaving them in isolation. The aim here is to provide you with adequate information and knowledge regarding all the influences that can affect your health, which relates to the restrictions, narrow-mindedness and injustices that take place within modern medicine and health care today. Some of these problems are due simply to human nature, but others are due to financial greed and the economics and politics of modern medicine. As this disease affects millions of women around the world then it is no surprise that many women will become caught up in this dysfunctional arena of medical 'care'.

What is Endometriosis?

We will first have a brief run-through of what endometriosis is, what the symptoms are and how it is diagnosed. The real truth is that doctors, scientists and researchers do not really know what is. They do know what the end results are, but these are not the same for every woman. This disease cannot be caught like other diseases, it is not sexually transmitted, and it is not a form of cancer.

Fundamentally, endometriosis is a chronic and serious physical malfunction, originating in the reproductive organs, striking millions of women in their most formative years. It is a complex disabling disease, with many symptoms, and has huge repercussions in a woman's' life.

The term endometriosis is derived from ancient Greek:

    endo means inside
    metra mean womb
    osis means disease or abnormality

Little progress has been made in the medical field in relation to endometriosis diagnosis or treatment - despite its importance as an increasing worldwide health problem. Most of the treatment available today revolves around the management of pain, drug intervention of the reproductive cycle and surgery to cut out the diseased tissue and remove adhesions that can occur in the abdomen.

There is currently no mainstream medical procedure that is guaranteed to remove the disease for good. In nearly all cases, after chemical or surgical intervention, there may be a short period of relief, but in many cases the disease returns.

This disease is fast becoming a scourge among females of childbearing age and beyond. Let's look at some statistics:

- It causes infertility in about 40 percent of its victims.
- There are over 5 million women and young girls in the US with this disease - and growing daily
- It is estimated that there are between 70 and 90 million women suffering with this disease worldwide.
- This estimated number of women suffering from endometriosis is based on a figure of 10% to 15% of women in their reproductive years. If the figure is only 10% of women who have it, that makes endometriosis one of the most common diseases on the face of the earth. More common than AIDS, more common than cancer
- Endometriosis accounts for more than 200,000 hysterectomies each year in the US alone – and rising
- The income generated for gynaecologists by endometriosis related hysterectomies in the US alone comes to roughly $288,000,000 per year. This is the cost for the operation only and does not include hospital costs.
- It can take on the average 9.28 years for a woman to get a diagnosis
- If you do a search on the Internet for Endometriosis at Google you get approximately 600,000 and growing. And yet so few people have heard of it. Why is that?

It is the invisible disease. All the symptoms are internal. There are no outward manifestations with it. Women do not walk around with a limp, or have to use crutches to get around, or have a serious rash, or have to use oxygen cylinders to aid breathing. There are simply no external physical clues.

Therefore most doctors dismiss these women as being hysterical, hypochondriacs, or it's 'all in the head'. It is only when women insist on further investigation due to relentless pain or serious problems with conception that they can then get to a specialist to look into her problems further. Even then, this disease can only be diagnosed for certain by having an investigative operation that physically allows the surgeon to see inside the woman's body. It is then and only then that all is revealed.

In some cases what can be found inside a woman's abdomen can look like a battlefield. There can be cysts all over the abdominal cavity, adhesions, and some of these adhesions can actually stick internal organs together. But for nearly every woman who is told that 'the cause of her problems have been found', this can be a huge relief. Simply because she now knows that there is a real and tangible reason why she has felt so awful and been in so much pain. She now knows what it is. She can start to find out about it and get herself informed. She can now take action for her own health - NOW THAT SHE KNOWS WHAT IT IS.

So what has happened physically inside a Womans' Body?

It is becoming more and more evident that this disease is either an autoimmune disease, or an Immune Deficiency disease, which for some reason focuses on the reproductive system, causing damage to the organs, damage to the immune system and untold damage to a woman's life.

Physical Changes

The womb is lined with tissue called the endometrium. Somehow, tiny particles of tissue, which are very similar to the endometrium, find their way to other regions of the body, but mainly in the pelvic cavity, where they attach to other organs.

It is not clear from medical research whether these particles are identical to the tissue in the lining of the womb or very similar and derived by some other mechanism. These tiny particles react to the monthly hormonal changes of the female reproductive cycle. So just as the normal endometrium tissue will fill with blood each month, in preparation for the development of an embryo, the abnormal particles in the abdominal cavity will behave in the same way.

Each month they react to hormones and breakdown and bleed. But there is nowhere for the blood to go during the normal shedding process of the menstrual cycle. So a woman has internal bleeding from the location of these particles. Gradually these particles develop into growths or lesions, which over time become bigger and bigger, as the monthly build up of blood has nowhere to go.

Another point that has conflicting findings in my research is the issue of whether the diseased particles or lesions in the abdomen do actual behave cyclically or not. Some authorities have found that the lesions can bleed at any time of the month, which would explain why some women have pain throughout the month.

The action of the bleeding from these abnormal endometrial sites causes pain and leads to scar tissue formation. Adhesions can develop causing organs to stick together. There is usually inflammation at the sites of the implants, bowel problems, ovulation pain and infertility in many cases.

The location of these growths are most commonly found on the ovaries, fallopian tubes, the ligaments that support the uterus, the area between the vagina and rectum called the Pouch of Douglas, the outer surface of the uterus and the lining of the pelvic cavity. These are the most common sites for endometriosis to be found, but it has also been found in other far distant locations of the body including the lungs, the eyes and the limbs. In fact endometriosis has been found in every organ of the body except the spleen.

The levels of pain experienced by women vary greatly, but on the whole most women have excruciating pain with this disease, especially around the time of their periods and during ovulation. Nearly all women with endometriosis suffer from other health problems which are probably due to the breakdown of the immune system.

Some of these are:

- Chronic fatigue syndrome
- Irritable bowel syndrome
- ME
- Food allergies
- Sleep problems (linked either to pain or hormonal imbalance)
- Yeast infections
- Susceptibility to infections (flu, colds etc)
- Depression

We will not go into any more detail here on the subject of what endometriosis is. You will already be aware from personal experience how devastating and far-reaching this disease can be. My role here is not to overwhelm you with lots of medical jargon.

There is a lot of information available about this disease, written from different viewpoints. If you require specific medical information then you need to go to your doctor, or check a medical information website or medical book. Also, there is a vast amount of advice and support you can gain from endometriosis message boards and support groups. You are well advised to get informed and find out as much as possible about this disease. Then you can make educated decisions as to how you wish to deal with it, how you wish your treatment programme to proceed, what questions you should be asking the medical profession, what conventional treatment options are available, what alternative options are available, and how you can help yourself.

To get informed about this disease many women use the Internet. I have used all sorts of words at search engines to do my research. As I said earlier, if you do a search for Endometriosis at Google there is enough advice there to last you a life. OK, some of these are duplicate results, but that is still an awful lot of information. My own search even took me as far as Greenpeace, which will be revealed later.

Add other words to your search, for example add the words 'side-effects' when looking up a particular drug treatment. You may be shocked at what you find. Getting as much information as possible is the only way you will understand this elusive disease. You may find contradictory advice, confusing advice, advice or factual information which is unclear; but believe me, the more you research this disease, sooner or later common threads begin to appear, and you will find further information that validates what you may have found elsewhere.

But the aim of this book is to try and steer you away from all the negative and scary stories about endometriosis. My intent is to be positive, and only to include enough background information to put this book and its contents into context.

Symptoms of Endometriosis

The symptoms of endometriosis can vary from nearly non-existent to incapacitating, but the women who have hardly any symptoms are very few indeed. On the whole women suffer from pelvic pain with their periods and with ovulation, and in some cases this pain can be so excruciating, with the need for some women to go to the emergency department of their local hospital, especially around the time of their period.

The most common symptom for women is the worsening of their menstrual cramps, becoming progressively worse as time goes by. Unfortunately many women are brought up to believe that it is normal to have painful periods. Pain can also occur throughout the month for some women.

The main symptoms associated with endometriosis
   Pain
   - painful periods
   - pain during and/or after sexual intercourse

- pelvic and/or abdominal pain (not necessarily at the time of menstruation)
- lower back pain
- ovulation pain
- thigh and/or leg pain
- pain during internal examination of the vagina and/or bowel

Bleeding problems
- heavy bleeding and/or clotting
- prolonged bleeding
- premenstrual spotting
- irregular bleeding
- irregular cycles

Bowel and bladder symptoms
- painful bowel movements
- pain when passing wind
- bowel pain
- diarrhoea and/or constipation
- bleeding from the bowel
- nausea and/or vomiting
- pain when passing urine
- urinary frequency

Other
- lethargy and/or malaise
- depression and/or irritability
- premenstrual syndrome (PMS)
- swollen abdomen
- insomnia

Pain is the predominant symptom for most women – sometimes this pain is associated with a woman's periods, but other women can suffer pain for most of the time.

Symptoms in Relation to areas of the Body

Reproductive Area Endometriosis

Pelvic pain

Pelvic pain is one of the most common symptoms of endometriosis. The pelvic pain of endometriosis can be excruciating and debilitating for many women. It may be experienced constantly, it may be intermittent or it may be related solely to the menstrual period. Pain can be provoked by certain activities such as walking, standing too long etc., or it may occur unpredictably.

Occasionally abdominal and pelvic pain may be caused by Irritable Bowel Syndrome (IBS). These two diseases are quite common together, so it is advised to take note of the times you experience pelvic pain, as it may coincide after meal times.

Lower Back Pain

Lower back pain is another common but poorly recognised symptom that often accompanies period pain. It is commonly associated with endometriosis in the Pouch of Douglas, uterosacral ligaments, and rectovaginal septum.

Ovulation Pain

Ovulation pain can occur in women who do not have endometriosis, but this pain will normally be a small twinge. In women with endometriosis, ovulation pain can be rather acute, and is another symptom of the disease. Pain usually begins 12-24 hours before ovulation and may last for a few days. It results from the normal enlargement of the ovary during ovulation which causes stretching of endometrial implants and adhesions lying on the surface of the ovary. The pain is often described as 'stabbing' and it may radiate throughout the pelvic area and into the buttocks and thighs.

The Main Reproductive Symptoms of Endometriosis are:

- Chronic or intermittent pelvic pain
- Ectopic (tubal) pregnancy
- Dysmenorrhea (painful menstruation is not normal!)
- Infertility
- Miscarriage(s)
- Painful ovulation

Uterosacral/Presacral Nerve Endometriosis:

- Backache
- Leg pain
- Painful Intercourse

Cul de Sac ('Pouch of Douglas') Endometriosis:

- Dyspareunia (pain during intercourse)
- Gastrointestinal symptoms
- Pain after intercourse

Gastrointestinal Endometriosis

(rectosigmoid colon, rectovaginal septum, small bowel, rectum, large bowel, appendix, gallbladder, intestinal tract)

The bowel symptoms of endometriosis are often overlooked or dismissed because many people think endometriosis affects only the reproductive organs. Many bowel symptoms are caused by irritation to the bowel from endometrial implants lying on adjacent areas such as the Pouch of Douglas and the back of the uterus, but some are due to endometrial deposits lying on the outside of the bowel wall.

One particular gastrointestinal disorder which is most common with endometriosis is Irritable Bowel Syndrome which can cause many of the bowel symptoms mentioned below. Candida has also been found to be prevalent in women with endometriosis, and this too can cause many distressing digestive upsets and discomfort.

The Main Gastrointestinal Symptoms of Endometriosis are:

- Nausea
- Diarrhoea

- Blood in stool
- Bloating
- Vomiting
- Rectal pain
- Rectal bleeding
- Tailbone pain
- Abdominal cramping
- Constipation
- Sharp gas pains
- Painful bowel movements

Endometriosis of the Bowel

A Further Explanation

Numerous women suffer with a range of upsetting symptoms of the bowel caused by endometriosis. Many gynaecologists and doctors are beginning to understand the relationship between bowel symptoms and endometriosis. However, too many doctors still do not think of endometriosis when their young female patients report symptoms such as intermittent constipation or diarrhoea, or alternating bouts of the two. Most importantly, they do not think to ask the young woman if her bowel symptoms vary with her menstrual cycle – the key feature of bowel symptoms due to endometriosis. As a result, some young women are not being diagnosed with endometriosis.

Causes

Most bowel symptoms are not due to the presence of endometriosis on the surface of the bowel itself. Rather, they are usually due to irritation from implants and nodules located in adjacent areas, such as the Pouch of Douglas, uterosacral ligaments, and rectovaginal septum.

In those cases where the endometrial implants are located on the bowel, the implants are usually lying on the outside surface of the bowel or rectum rather than in the bowel itself. Nevertheless, endometriosis can penetrate into and through the bowel wall on some occasions. The large bowel is a much more common site of endometriosis than the small bowel. Some bowel symptoms are due to adhesions constricting, twisting, or pulling on the bowel.

Diagnosis

Diagnosing bowel symptoms due to endometriosis relies a great deal on the woman's description of her symptoms and menstrual history. Bowel symptoms due to endometriosis are generally only present or are worse around the time of the period, though they may be present throughout the month. They are also usually reported along with one or more of the classical symptoms of endometriosis, such as painful periods and painful intercourse, rather than on their own.

Women whose bowel symptoms are due to endometrial nodules in the Pouch of Douglas may find a vaginal examination painful. The gynaecologist may also be able to feel nodules in the Pouch of Douglas.

Sometimes the gynaecologist will refer the woman to a bowel specialist if he or she is not sure whether the bowel symptoms are due to endometriosis or another cause. Occasionally, the gynaecologist may refer the woman to a bowel specialist for a colonoscopy. A colonoscopy is an examination of the inside of the bowel with a telescope-like instrument. In most women with endometriosis, the colonoscopy will be normal because endometrial implants and nodules rarely penetrate through the wall of the bowel wall so they are not visible during a colonoscopy.

Treatment

Endometrial nodules in the Pouch of Douglas, uterosacral ligaments, and rectovaginal septum are generally larger and deeper than ordinary implants. They do not usually respond to drug treatment so they will usually be removed surgically. Because they are difficult to reach, there is a danger that the bowel may be damaged accidentally during surgery. Therefore, the surgeon must be experienced at laparoscopic surgery.

Cutting (excision) techniques are usually used rather than burning techniques. Superficial endometrial implants on the surface of the bowel are usually removed by carefully removing the relevant part of the membrane that covers the bowel wall.

If the endometriosis has penetrated through a section of the bowel wall that section of the bowel may have to be removed (bowel resection). Few gynaecologists are able to perform bowel resections, so usually a bowel surgeon will be called in to perform the resection.

Other Locations & Symptoms of Endometriosis

Urinary Tract (Urethra) Endometriosis

The urinary tract symptoms of endometriosis are usually the result of endometriosis lying on the outside of the bladder or irritation from endometrial implants lying on the front of the uterus.

The Main Symptoms of Urinary Tract Endometriosis are:

- Blood in urine
- Painful or burning urination
- Hypertension
- Tenderness around the kidneys
- Flank pain radiating toward the groin
- Urinary frequency, retention, or urgency

Pleural (Lung and Chest Cavity) Endometriosis

Very occasionally endometriosis can travel to the lungs, which will give rise to strange symptoms, and are usually relate to the menstrual cycle.

- Coughing up of blood or bloody sputum, particularly coinciding with menses
- Accumulation of air or gas in the chest cavity
- Constricting chest pain and/or shoulder pain
- Collection of blood and/or pulmonary nodule in chest cavity (revealed under testing)
- Shortness of breath

Sciatic Endometriosis

- Pain in the leg and/or hip which radiates down the leg (this symptom is concurrent with that of inguinal Endometriosis - groin area - as well.

Skin Endometriosis

- Painful nodules, often visible to the naked eye, at the skin's surface. Can bleed during menses and/or appear blue upon inspection.

Dyspareunia (Painful Intercourse)

Dyspareunia is a common symptom of endometriosis. Pain may be felt during intercourse as well as up to 48 hours after sexual activity. It is often associated with endometriosis in the pouch of Douglas or adhesions in the pelvic cavity. Intercourse can also disturb endometrial patches or scar tissue in the pelvic area.

Fatigue

Fatigue and endometriosis seem to go hand in hand. No one knows what causes the acute fatigue women suffer with this disease, and is not often recognised as a symptom of endometriosis.

Fatigue can be one of the most debilitating aspects of the disease, and most women with endometriosis experience fatigue around the time of their period and some experience it throughout the month. The fatigue may be related to the constant pain and/or medication, or it could be the bodies' reaction to the disease at a deeper level.

Abdominal Bloating

Abdominal bloating may be a symptom of endometriosis. It is thought to be due to inflammation in the pelvic cavity caused by the endometriosis. As mentioned above, Irritable Bowel Syndrome (IBS) can cause pelvic pain, and can also cause severe abdominal bloating. With IBS, the bloating is usually caused by intestinal gasses which expand and distend the abdomen and can cause severe pain and discomfort. IBS is very common in women with endometriosis.

Stages of Endometriosis

Mild endometriosis - implants are small, flat patches of endometrial tissue growing outside of their normal location.

Moderate endometriosis - includes "chocolate cysts" of endometriosis may be smaller than a pea or larger than a grapefruit, located within the ovary.

Severe endometriosis - in some cases, bands of fibrous scar tissues (adhesions) bind the pelvic organs together.

Interestingly enough, except for the obvious mechanical obstruction found in severe endometriosis, there seems to be no real correlation between the severity of endometriosis and its impact on fertility. However, as many as half of the women who have been diagnosed with infertility are found to have endometriosis on laparoscopic examination

Usually speaking, the more advanced the disease the worse the pain becomes. But this is not always the case. For some women microscopic lesions may cause huge amounts of pain, whereas another woman who has much larger lesions may have little discomfort. But for most women chronic pelvic pain becomes evident most of the time. If the intestines are involved, then cyclic bowel changes may occur, causing painful defecation and sometimes rectal bleeding.

These are the main symptoms that are most common with endometriosis. They are the localised symptoms relating to the damage in the abdominal cavity caused by endometriosis. But because the immune system is compromised then other problems sometimes develop like ME and Chronic Fatigue Syndrome.

Because the symptoms of endometriosis are so inconsistent, non-specific and can vary from one woman to another, it can easily resemble other conditions including appendicitis, ovarian cysts, a bowel construction, colon cancer, fibroid tumours, irritable bowel syndrome, and pelvic inflammatory disease. This is why it is so important for a woman to get a correct diagnosis.

Diagnosis of Endometriosis

Obtaining a diagnosis for this disease can be one of the most difficult things to achieve. There are many possible reasons for this including:

- lack of knowledge or awareness of the disease among the medical profession, despite the growing numbers of women who have this disease world-wide
- the obvious lack of knowledge about the disease by the women themselves because there is a lack of public awareness, so women are unable to find out about it - catch 22
- a woman's symptoms being wrongly diagnosed, and most commonly diagnosed as pelvic inflammatory disease
- many women think that their symptoms are normal and do not suspect that anything is wrong until it progressively gets worse over time. So there is a delay in getting their disease diagnosed which means that more damage has been done
- most patients found information on endometriosis in magazines and from friends rather than their doctors
- many women are not taken seriously by their doctors even when they describe the severity of their symptoms

As mentioned earlier, getting a diagnosis can be very difficult because the symptoms of endometriosis resemble other gynaecological problems. During a physical examination your doctor may find nodules in the back of the vagina, in the rectum and on the ligaments supporting the uterus. The ovaries may be tender and enlarged, there could be lumps in the abdomen or the uterus drawn back and attached to the rectum. But finding these changes in the abdomen cannot tell the doctor if the patient has endometriosis, pelvic growths, pelvic inflammatory disease or any other condition that causes anatomical changes.

It is now agreed that the only safe and reliable way to determine what is wrong is for a woman to have a laparoscopy. During laparoscopic surgery, a small lighted telescope is inserted into a tiny incision near the navel, so the organs can be seen. It is during this procedure that the evidence of endometriosis can be seen, usually with cysts and adhesions in the pelvic cavity. The actual true diagnosis is done by a biopsy, using a sample of the endometriosis growths. *(Details of a Laparoscopy procedure are covered later on.)*

Other procedures, such as ultrasound scans, barium enemas with x-ray, computed tomography, and magnetic resonance imaging (MRI), may be used to determine the extent of the disease and follow its course, but their usefulness in diagnosis is limited.

Once a diagnosis has been made a woman can then take action to find out more about the disease. She will be able to make informed decisions as to how she wants to deal with it and be able to find other sufferers and get their advice and support.

Getting the Best from your Doctor/Physician

When discussing your health with a doctor or physician it is advised to be prepared for your appointment. Start to write down the questions you want to ask well before hand. If you leave it to ask questions as you think of them at your appointment, you will easily forget to ask about some crucial or important advice.

How to prepare:

- Think clearly about your symptoms and how they affect your life
- Make a list of all your symptoms
- Better still, try to keep a diary and then write up the details. Take this list with you and read them out
- Rehearse what you are going to say beforehand, wither with someone else or just in your own mind
- Take someone with you to the consultation for support. Sometimes we can be overcome by too many emotions to convey clearly what we want to know, and having someone else there will help to keep the focus.
- If you think you need longer than usual with your doctor then book a double appointment.
- Take with you the names of any drugs or medicines you have been taking to help with the symptoms. If you write up in your diary when you are taking pain medication, this helps to strengthen the case of how severely your health is affected.
- If the doctor suggests a physical examination, ask them what sort of information this might give.
- If there is anything you do not understand, ask your doctor to explain - as many times as is necessary!
- If you are prescribed any drugs, ask if there are any side effects you should look out for.
- Ask how much experience your doctor has had in treating endometriosis and how much they understand about the disease. If your doctor does not know very much about endometriosis then you are advised to change to another doctor. You need informed and sympathetic advice for this disease, not guesswork or token gestures for treatment simply to get you out of the door.

Test for Endometriosis

The only reliable way to diagnose endometriosis is to actually see it during an operation. However, there are other tests which you might undergo before being referred for a laparoscopy.

Physical examination:

During physical examination the doctor is looking for indications of possible endometriosis, such as pelvic mass (where organs feel as though they are matted together with scar tissue) which feel tender. Evidence of large cysts may be checked out as well. A physical examination may include:

- Feeling your abdomen on the outside to see if there is any tenderness, or if lumps can be felt through the abdominal wall muscles.
- Doing an internal examination to check that the vagina, womb and ovaries are not tender or affected by lumps.
- Examining the rectum to check the ligaments (muscle bands of strong tissue) to see if there are any lumps behind the womb.

It is important to remember that if the outcome of these examinations is that everything seems normal, is does not mean that you do not have endometriosis. You may be asked to come back another time, because some problems do not show up until mid-cycle or just before or during your period.

Imaging techniques:

The ultrasound scan is the main imaging technique used. It is completely harmless and is exactly the same devise as is used to scan pregnant women. Some gel is put on your stomach and a scanning head is then passed over your abdomen. It works by passing high-frequency sound waves through the body, which is then bounced back to form an image of your pelvic organs on a computer screen.

The problems with this type of diagnosis is that it cannot distinguish between the different types of pelvic mass detected (i.e.) whether it has found and endometrial deposit, a cyst or a tumour) and that it can only show up deposits of over two centimetres in size. So it is not a very reliable method to check and diagnose endometriosis.

Future tests:

Studies are still being carried out to develop a foolproof blood test which would reveal whether a woman has endometriosis. It has already been discovered that women with endometriosis have a raised amount of a substance called CA125 in their blood, which is secreted by endometrial tissue. The problem is that this substance is also secreted by other women (such as those who are pregnancy or have ovarian cancer). So it is impossible to tell without further investigation which condition is causing the rise.

Research is still underway to develop this test further so that it can be used in the future to detect endometriosis more clearly. This would allow for a diagnosis without the radical intervention of surgery.

Treatment of Endometriosis

Initial Thoughts

During the research for this book, the issue of treatment for endometriosis was the main topic where it was repeated again and again that there is no cure for Endometriosis. But there were certain places were I found seriously incorrect information on this subject. One source said, and I quote…………

'Definitive Surgical Therapy.' This is the only cure for endometriosis and involves hysterectomy with removal of ovaries (oophorectomy) along with endometrial implants.'

The facts are that women can still have recurring endometriosis even after removal of the womb and ovaries. A woman can still have recurring endometriosis after menopause. There is more on this later. The above quote comes from a sizeable, and no doubt reputable and profitable, training and health care provider based in California.

This is why information about this disease has to be broadcast, and soon. There will be many women, who are undergoing major surgery to remove all their reproductive organs in the hope of getting rid of endometriosis. It is simply not the case. When you look at the income generated for gynaecologist in the US with regard to endometriosis related hysterectomies, I start to smell a rat here! This disease is making big bucks for some people. We will go more into this matter later as well.

The financial situation is not the same in the UK as there is a national health service, providing free health care to all citizens, and there is similar provision in other countries in Europe. But for women who have to pay for their health care, the cost of treatment can be a huge burden.

Treatment Options

There are a range of treatments available to women with endometriosis within mainstream medicine. In most cases a woman will have been referred to a gynaecologist for her treatment, and usually a definite diagnosis will have been done with the laparoscopy.

Due to the limited knowledge or experience of this disease in the medical profession, the objective of the treatment offered today, is to help relieve the pain and reduce the symptoms. Treatment also aims to shrink or slow down the endometrial growths, to try and restore fertility and to delay the recurrence of the disease.

A woman's treatment should be decided in partnership between her and her medical advisors. If you do decide to pursue your treatment with orthodox medicine, there will be a number of factors to take into account when deciding which treatment path to follow. This will include:

- Severity and type of symptoms - may influence your options of treatment. Some women with endometriosis have little or no symptoms; and no treatment may be needed. If symptoms are mild, painkillers alone may be sufficient. Hormone treatments are sometimes effective at easing pain but do not improve fertility. Surgery may be suggested if infertility is caused by endometriosis.
- Age and plans for pregnancy - symptoms often improve during pregnancy. The longer you have endometriosis the greater the chance that it will reduce your fertility. Also, the longer you leave endometriosis unchecked, the more damage it will do, and the more pain it will cause.
- Success of treatment and side effects - the hormone treatment options all have similar success rates at easing pain, but they all have side effects. Some of these side effects are intolerable by some women and so treatment may be switched from one drug to another.
- Recurrences - once endometriosis has been cleared with a course of treatment it may recur again in the future. In fact, in most cases it does recur. A new course of hormone treatment and/or surgery will have to be contemplated. I have read cases where some women have had up to 20 surgical procedures due to this disease.
- Personal choice - a woman should choose for herself which treatment option to take. She should not be coerced into any one type of treatment because it is the easiest for the physician, or it is the specialism of the physician. It is also advisable to get a second opinion. You may get 2 totally different approaches and attitudes to this disease and its treatment. One physician may be counting his days to retirement and the other physician may have some personal experience of the disease. You need to feel at ease with you chosen health care provider no matter which field of medicine they work in. This goes along way to having faith in the process of healing. This subject is covered in more detail later on.

Pain Medication

There are various over-the-counter pain relief drugs that can be used for endometriosis. In some case prescription drugs may be required if the pain is very severe. There are also a number of non-steroid anti-inflammatory drugs (NSAIDs) used to help relieve pain. Narcotic painkillers such as codeine, and morphine, as well as narcotics combined with other pain relief drugs may also be prescribed.

Problems with Painkillers

Women with endometriosis do not find the over-the-counter drugs very effective, especially as they seem to be less effective over time. It is not effective to take stringer painkillers, as prescribed by your doctor, for too long as they can become addictive. It may be advisable to switch between different strengths of painkillers to suit different levels of pain. For instance, reserve the very strong ones when your pain is worse with your periods.

What are the Side Effects of Painkillers?

All painkillers can irritate the stomach lining, cause nausea and vomiting and in some cases lead to coughing up blood. Quite often they cause constipation or diarrhoea.

Over the Counter Painkillers

Paracetamol - this acts as a painkiller but it does not have anti-inflammatory properties. It is probably the easiest painkiller to take and has fewer side effects than other analgesics (medical term for painkillers). However, paracetamol may be less effective for more mild pain.

Aspirin - reduces inflammation and fever, but can cause stomach irritation so should not be taken with food or milk. It is good for mild to moderate pain.

Ibuprofen - another popular anti-inflammatory. It has a mild painkilling effect but it can also irritate the stomach.

NSAIDs

NSAIDs are a class of drugs which are designed to relieve pain as well as reduce inflammation. These drugs may vary in degrees of analgesic versus anti-inflammatory activity. This means that one drug may have a great deal of anti-inflammatory properties but little in the way of pain reduction help; whereas another drug may primarily be a painkiller with little ability to reduce inflammation. They can be bought over-the-counter, though some stronger versions are only available on prescription.

NSAIDs stands for 'Non-steroidal anti-inflammatory drug', and are available under various trade names. As well as having some painkilling action they also work by inhibiting the production of prostaglandins in the body.

Prostaglandins are chemicals made by body tissues; they send messages to the womb causing it to shrink, and also cause the womb-walls to contract during periods or childbirth. They are also part of the body's natural healing mechanism, as they go to the sites of injury and activate its pain receptors, causing inflammation. It is thought endometriosis sufferers have extra prostaglandins because these can be produced by endometriosis tissue.

The idea behind NSAIDs is that if you introduce drugs which block prostaglandins, you will suffer less pain. They work best if they are taken early in the pain-cycle. For instance, if you know you usually experience pain on Day 21 of your cycle, it is a good idea to start taking them the previous day.

Prescribed Painkillers

Your doctor may prescribe stronger painkillers if over-the-counter painkillers are not strong enough.

Mild to moderate strength - co-analgesics, which are a mixture of codeine and paracetamol.

Moderate to strong - dihydrocodeine, also known as DF118, and nefopan are both moderate to strong painkillers, but can cause constipation and dependency.

Strongest - opiates or opoids, such as morphine and pethidine. These are only prescribed for severe pain and are not suitable for long-term use as you can become dependent quickly, even at low doses.

Hormone Treatments

There are several different types of drugs used for the treatment of endometriosis. The main aim of all of them is to stop you having periods for six to nine months. The theory is that once hormones released before or during your period no longer stimulate the patches of endometriosis, these patches will shrink and stop causing pain.

Understanding how hormone treatments work

Estrogen is a hormone that is made mainly in the ovaries. It is also produced in other parts of the body in small amounts, but it is the ovaries that make the most. Estrogen is needed by the cells lining the inside of the uterus (endometrial cells) to make them grow and survive. The endometrial cells found outside the womb that cause endometriosis also need estrogen to survive. As mentioned earlier, it is not clear in the medical authorities whether the cells that cause endometriosis are identical to the cells in the lining of the womb (endometrium), or whether these cells are just very similar. Whatever the case, they do react to estrogen just the same.

The stimulus to make estrogen comes from hormones called gonadotrophins. These are made in the pituitary gland next to the brain. These in turn are caused to be released into the bloodstream by a hormone from higher in the brain called gonadotrophin-releasing hormone (or GnRH for short).

Hormone treatment aims to stop estrogen from being made or to block its effects on the endometrial cells. The endometrial cells are then starved of the estrogen which normally makes them grow and survive. Therefore, patches of endometriosis gradually shrink and may clear up.

Which Drug Treatment to Take?

Personally I do not advocate the use of hormone drug treatment for endometriosis. But should you decide on this option you need to get as much advice from your doctor if you are to try the drug treatment route. Obviously the best drug to take is the one which is the most effective for you and has the fewest side effects. The side effects vary from person to person, and the only way to find out would be to take the drug for a while to see how it affects you.

Most drug treatment programmes are for six-month periods, but you will be asked to return to your doctor to monitor your progress and find out how you are getting on. If you have any serious side effects, you are advised to stop treatment immediately and report these to your doctor. This includes raised blood pressure, tightness in your chest or any other symptoms you find intolerable.

Drugs used in Hormone Treatment Include:

Testosterone Derivatives

Danazol - a synthetic form of the male hormone (testosterone) which induces a pseudo-menopause. This drug acts on the pituitary gland and stops it from secreting the natural hormones required for ovulation. In turn it drastically reduces the ovaries' production of estrogen and progesterone to an amount too small to support monthly periods. Treatment may last from 3 to 9 months in which time it allows the endometrial growths to shrink, and will alleviate the pain related to menstruation.

As well as being used to relieve pain, it is also prescribed for a short term prior to surgery to reduce and shrink endometrial deposits to make surgery easier.

Progestogen Hormone Tablets

Progesterone is a female hormone responsible for preparing the womb for pregnancy. In its synthetic form it can cause the womb lining to shrink and, along with it, any other endometrial deposits. 'Progestogen is basically the name given to any substance which has the same effects as the natural hormone Progesterone. Progestogens trick the body into thinking it is pregnant, resulting in lowering of the levels of estrogen in the body which helps relieve endometriosis.

Progesterone hormone tablets - oppose the estrogen effects on the endometrial growths which cause them to 'shrink'. Progesterone also prevents ovulation which lowers the estrogen levels. Side effects include: irregular menstrual bleeding, weight gain, mood changes, bloating, fatigue, depression, and nausea.

You should stop taking Progesterone treatment if you suffer any of the following: migraines, pain or tightness of the chest, high blood pressure, itching, and jaundice.

It has long been known that progestogens can alter the blood lipids (fats) in an unfavourable way, which might theoretically lead to an increased risk of blood clots (thrombosis). Two recent studies have provided more evidence that this could be the case. Although they looked at progestogens used for period problems, the doses used are similar as would be for treatment of endometriosis, and the risk of thrombosis was around 5-fold higher than expected

Progestogen hormone drugs for Endometriosis include:

    Medroxyprogesterone (Provera)
    Norethisterone (Primolut)
    Dydrogesterone (Duphaston)

Gestrinone

Gestrinone is a synthetic hormone which has several different hormone actions with characteristics of both male and female hormones. It is not fully understood how gestrinone works (so that should give you confidence!), but it seems to act in two ways:

- It suppresses the release of the FSH and LH from the pituitary gland. Without this stimulation of the ovaries, ovulation usually stops thus preventing the growth of endometriosis.

- It also seems directly to suppress the endometriosis deposits

As it lasts a long time in the body, gestrinone only needs to be taken twice a week

GnRH Analogues

Gonadotropin releasing hormone - analogues are classified into 2 groups: agonists and antagonist. Agonists are commonly used in the treatment of endometriosis by suppressing the manufacture of FSH and LH, common hormones required in ovulation. When they are not secreted, the body will go into pseudo-menopause. Ovulation ceases to take place with these drugs and near menopausal state results. This stops menstruation and the growth of endometrial tissue. These analogues commonly cause side effects in most women (see below).

GnRH analogues cannot be given by mouth, at they break down too quickly before having any effect. So they are usually taken in the form of nasal sprays, slow-release implants or as an intra-muscular injection.

The side effects can be relieved, by adding back estrogen and progesterone, which does not affect the benefit of treatment. This is known as Add-Back therapy for endometriosis. One of the GnRH drugs which are commonly prescribed is known as Lupron. There is a lot of information about this drug on the Internet, as well as lots of mention of it at endometriosis chat groups. This drug is also used for other health problems in both men and women. So it is not designed specifically for the treatment of endometriosis, and some women have found they now have serious long-term health problems caused by this drug.

GnRH drugs used to treat Endometriosis include:

Leuprorelin (Prostap)
Goserelin (Zoladex)
Nafarelin (Synarel)
Buserelin (Suprecur)
Lupron

Warnings of Lupron

As mentioned above, the hormone drug treatment of Lupron is gaining a very bad reputation, with much bad press. This has culminated in many legal cases, where women have taken the manufacturers to court because of the serious damage it has caused to the health of these women.

Up to the spring of 1999, the FDA had received 4228 reports of adverse drug events from women using Lupron™ (Interestingly, they also received 2943 such reports from men, who used the drug in prostate cancer treatment, and despite the differences in age, sex, and indication for use, the complaints were remarkably similar) 325 adverse events reported for women resulted in hospitalisation, and additionally, 25 deaths were reported. Whether these deaths are directly attributable to Lupron remains to be determined, and the FDA has indicated that it does not have enough staff to follow up on this matter now.

A few years late there followed a lawsuit against the manufacturers of Lupron which resulted in many successful claims for damages to long-term health.

Oral Contraceptives

The combined oral contraceptive pill is often used in the treatment of endometriosis. There are many different brands of the Pill on the market. This treatment approach is usually the first to be suggested for the treatment of endometriosis. It is one way to 'buy time' and to help relieve pain.

The combined contraceptive pill is basically made up of different combinations of synthetic estrogen and progesterone, which has the effect of mimicking pregnancy, causing the lining of the womb, along with endometrial deposits to shrink. When used to treat endometriosis, it is usually taken continuously. It is recommended to take low estrogen or progesterone only pill, because estrogen dominance will encourage further development of the endometrial growths.

It is often prescribed to teenagers and young women with a mild form of the disease, and sometimes to women who have recurring ovarian cysts.

Who can't take it?

- women with high blood pressure
- women who are at risk of developing blood clots
- smokers and women over the age of 35 are more at risk if the take the Pill over a long period of time.

The BCP (Birth Control Pill) is usually taken continuously for four to six months without the usual seven-day break which you have when taking it for contraceptive purposes. The success of the BCP for treatment of endometriosis is not as effective as with other hormone drug treatment. Many women find they have problems with break-through bleeding on the BCP, and some say it does not get rid of the pain.

Drugs Commonly used to Treat Endometriosis and their Side Effects

Drug	Side Effects
Combination oral contraceptive	Abdominal swelling, breast tenderness, increased appetite, ankle swelling, nausea, deep vain thrombosis.
Progesterone	Bleeding between periods, mood swings, depression, weight gain, fatigue, nausea, headaches, dizziness, bloating.
Danazol	Weight gain, acne, lowered voice, hair growth, hot flashes, vaginal dryness, ankle swelling, muscle cramps, decreased breast size, mood swings, liver malfunction, carpal tunnel syndrome, gastrointestinal upset.
Gestrinone	Muscle cramps, acne, breast shrinkage, fluid retention, itching, oily skin/hair.
GnRH agonists	Hot flashes, vaginal dryness, calcium loss from bone, mood swings, depression, loss of libido, sleep disturbance.

The Mirena Coil

Some doctors to treat the symptoms of endometriosis by reducing the amount of blood flow in a woman's periods use the Mirena Coil. The Mirena Coil is like many other types of Intrauterine Contraceptive Devices (IUD's or coils) in that it is fitted by a doctor and remains in the womb for a fixed amount of time, after which it must be changed.

Most IUD's make a woman's periods heavier, but the Mirena actually makes periods lighter than usual. Because of this, it is frequently used as a treatment for heavy periods, and is now used as a treatment option for endometriosis, for the same reason of reducing blood loss with the menstrual cycle.

It is made of a light, plastic T-shaped frame with the stem of the 'T' a bit thicker than the rest. This stem contains a tiny storage system of a hormone called Levonorgestrel. This hormone is also used in contraceptive pills. In the Mirena, however, a much lower dose is released than the Pill (about 1/7th strength), and it goes directly to the lining of the womb, rather than through the blood stream where it may lead to the common progesterone-type side effects.

Although the IUD was originally developed as a contraceptive, the discovery that it leads to much lighter periods was seen as a bonus. Many gynaecologists now suggest the Mirena as a treatment for heavy periods if tablet treatment doesn't work.

After 3 months use, the average blood loss is 85% less, and by 12 months the flow is reduced by 97% every cycle. About one third of women using the IUD will not have any periods at all. There is no 'build up' of blood, because the hormone in the IUD prevents the lining of the womb from building up at all.

Negatives of the Mirena Coil

There are many who feel that the Mirena Coil is very unsuitable as a treatment for endometriosis as this particular type of Coil increases the risk of developing ovarian cysts.

It is the use of synthetic Progestogen hormones used in the coil that increase the chance of benign ovarian cysts. This is more common with the higher hormone levels associated with the Progestogen-only pill. Overall the risk is about 3 times higher. The device could also lead to other complications of infection in the womb.

Surgery

There are different levels of surgery, and different approaches to surgery for the treatment of endometriosis, based mainly on the severity of the disease as well as the training and experience of your surgeon.

The decision whether or not to have surgery needs careful consideration, as all surgery and anaesthetic involves risk. Surgery is often used after a course of hormone drug treatment. The aim of the drugs is to make the endometrial growths and deposits reduce in size, making the surgical procedure easier.

Conservative surgery: this is when patches of endometrial tissue, cysts and adhesions are removed leaving your organs intact. The operational procedures for this type of surgery are varied and include Laparoscopy, Laparotomy, Laser Laparotomy and Microsurgery.

Radical surgery: is used to describe extensive surgery, and for Endometriosis this involves Hysterectomy of various types to remove some or all of the reproductive organs.

Why have Surgery?

There are various situations why surgery for the treatment of endometriosis may be needed including:

- drug treatment has not proved sufficient to reduce the disease
- your symptoms have returned after a course of drug treatment
- reconstruction of organs may be needed as treatment for infertility
- your endometriosis is severe, and includes adhesions and is affecting other important organs such as the bowel or intestines. (Surgery to your intestines and bowel carries risks as further damage can be caused to these organs during surgery.)

What are the advantages of surgery?

- surgery is seen as the only way to remove large or deeply embedded endometrial growths, cysts and adhesions
- surgery can sometimes restore the structure of the reproductive organs to help restore fertility
- some women do gain immediate relief for the pain of endometriosis after surgery, but in many cases the pain and symptoms return
- Laparoscopy is the only definitive method of obtaining a true diagnosis for this disease

What are the disadvantages of surgery?

- having and anaesthetic always carries risks
- the surgeon can only remove those endometriosis deposits which can be seen, so microscopic deposits can't be removed
- it is sometimes difficult to recognise endometriosis during surgery
- the endometriosis may be too close to sensitive organs, such as the bowel, and cannot be removed for fear of damaging the organ
- surgery might cause further adhesions
- endometriosis may still recur

Laparoscopy

Laparoscopy is the most common surgical procedure for the diagnosis and treatment of Endometriosis.

Laparoscopy is a relatively minor operation when used purely for diagnosis. It is when surgical treatment for endometriosis is done during a Laparoscopy that the procedure becomes more invasive and would be defined as major surgery.

A Laparoscopy is usually done under general anaesthetic. This type of operation may also be known as keyhole surgery, and is one of the lesser forms of invasive surgical treatment available today. There are some hospitals that will perform a Laparoscopy as an outpatient procedure, with the patient going home the same day. Many hospitals require the patient to stay over night, which allows for post surgery recovery to be monitored.

How is a Laparoscopy Performed?

A Laparoscopy is performed by first inflating the abdomen with gas, which is usually carbon dioxide, through a small incision near the navel. A long thin instrument called a Laparoscope is then carefully inserted into the inflated abdominal cavity to insect the abdomen and pelvis.

During surgery your body will be tilted slightly with the feet raised higher than the head. This allows some of the abdominal organs to shift upward toward the chest and out of the way. The gas that is used to inflate the abdomen helps to provide a better view inside the abdomen by pushing the abdominal wall and the bowel away from the organs in the pelvic cavity. This makes it easier for the surgeon to see the reproductive organs.

The laparoscope is a slender tube, like a miniature telescope, that is inserted through the small incision just below the navel. It is equipped with a lens for a clear view. A special attachment transmits light down through the tube, into the abdomen, so that the surgeon can see the ovaries, fallopian tubes and nearby organs.

Once the procedure is completed, the instruments are removed, the gas is released, and the incisions are closed. A few small stitches are usually placed to close the incision and the wound is dressed.

Laparoscopy used for Diagnosis of Endometriosis

During a Laparoscopic procedure, endometrial implants can be easily seen once these implants have reached a reasonable size. The implants that are still tiny cannot be seen by the naked eye. For an accurate diagnosis of endometriosis, small biopsies should be obtained during laparoscopy. A biopsy is the removal of tiny tissue samples for examination under a microscope. Some biopsies will show that endometriosis is evident, even though no endometrial implants are actually visible during the laparoscopy. This is why it is important to have a biopsy done when you have a laparoscopy, because some endometrial implants can be microscopic.

Laparoscopy for Treatment of Endometriosis

The same procedure for the diagnosis of endometriosis is used during surgical treatment of endometriosis. Your surgeon may go ahead and use further surgical techniques to treat endometrial implants during the first operation that has confirmed the diagnosis of endometriosis.

This usually requires the need for a second small incision in the abdomen so that additional surgical instruments can be inserted. These instruments will be used to surgically treat endometrial implants in a variety of ways. The technique being used by your surgeon depends on various factors including:

- training for different procedures
- experience of different procedures
- type of equipment being used

For the surgical treatment of endometriosis, your surgeon will aim to remove endometrial implants, separate any adhesions, and drain and treat any large cysts.

Laparoscopic surgery requires the use of various instruments to perform different repairs to any damaged tissue and organs caused by endometriosis. Diathermy, which uses an electric current, may be used to divide tissue as well as coagulate tissue, particularly blood vessels to control any bleeding. Light energy in the form of lasers may also be used. Laser treatment can be used to 'burn' endometrial cysts and to cut away adhesions. The advantage of laser surgery is that the effectiveness of the laser is very precise and reduces tissue damage.

Length of Operation

This will depend on what treatment is performed. If you are having your first laparoscopy with the aim of obtaining a diagnosis, then the laparoscopy usually takes between 20 to 30 minutes. If further treatment is performed to deal with endometrial growths and adhesions, it may last up to an hour.

To Sum Up

Laparoscopic surgery when performed successfully, affords much less postoperative discomfort and a faster recovery than conventional surgery. Surgical techniques and equipment have developed greatly in the last few decades. Any form of surgery carries risks, and any form of trauma to the body will cause pain and postoperative reactions.

Laser Laparoscopy

Laser Laparoscopy refers to various types of laser equipment which are used when performing a Laparoscopy. The word laser is an abbreviation for light amplification by stimulated emission of radiation. Various substances give out a very thin beam of light when they are stimulated by an electric charge. This beam of light can then be controlled using mirrors, and directed down a laparoscope very precisely on to one area to burn away or vaporise endometrial tissue. These lasers are so accurate that it is possible for them to cut grooves into human hair. Because they are so precise, they cause no damage to surrounding tissues during treatment.

There are four main types of laser:

- the carbon dioxide laser - used for treating mild to moderate endometriosis because it is easy to control
- the argon laser - for vaporising large cysts and sealing blood vessels
- the KTP (potassium titabyl phosphate) laser - penetrates deeply and is effective for treating large, deeply embedded cysts which are difficult to get at
- the YAG (neodymium - yttrium aluminium garnet) laser - used to destroy large deposits because it penetrates deeply into tissue

What happens during laser laparoscopy?

As well as the two usual cuts which are made during a laparoscopy (through which the laparoscope and the handling instruments are passed) two more tiny incisions are made on either side of the abdomen (though this may vary from one surgeon to another), below the bikini line. One is for the laser and the other for the venting devise which allows waste-gases and tissue out of the abdomen, and through which fluid is passed to wash out the cavity. The laser is then used to divide adhesions, vaporise deposits of endometriosis, drain cysts and improve fertility by reconstructive surgery.

What are the advantages of laser laparoscopy?

- laser burns heal very quickly with minimum scar tissue and bleeding
- it has a 70% success rate in relieving abdominal pain
- it can greatly increase your chances of pregnancy because it is less invasive while doing repair work to your reproductive organs
- the treatment is more accurate than conventional surgical techniques

Note: Laser laparoscopy does not increase chances of your surgeon finding all the endometrial implants and deposits, so the risk of endometriosis returning are the same as with conventional surgery - but healing is quicker and there is much less risk of adhesions being caused by the actual operation.

Laparotomy

A Laparotomy is a major operation to open the abdomen, remove endometrial sites and correct any other problems with the reproductive organs. This operation is not as popular now with the development of the Laparoscopy.

This procedure is done when the endometriosis is more extensive and involves more of the abdominal cavity. It involves opening up the abdominal cavity because the work cannot be done through a tiny incision as used in laparoscopy. When endometriosis has affected the appendix, bladder, bowel or kidney, for example, it may require special surgical techniques only practised with Laparotomy. This procedure requires a longer stay in hospital and a longer recovery time.

Some of the reasons why you may have a Laparotomy are:

- there were complications during a Laparoscopy
- you suffer from severe endometriosis and adhesions
- there is a need to do more extensive surgical work on other organs
- you are overweight, which can make a Laparoscopy difficult

What happens during a Laparotomy?

After a general anaesthetic, a 10 to 15 cm cut is made below the bikini line. Any endometrial cysts and patches are removed, and adhesions are separated and removed if possible. Various surgical instruments are used to perform the different procedures during the operation.

This type of operation is more invasive firstly due to the larger opening through the abdominal wall, and trauma to the abdominal cavity may be greater due to the amount of work your surgeon may need to do. The operation may take longer, which requires being under anaesthetic for longer.

Microsurgery

Microsurgery is a relatively new technique which involves special teflon-coated metal tools which do not cause abrasions and adhesions because of their non-stick surface. Incisions are made with a hot wire which cuts as well as seals, and the 'debris' is then removed by suction. The procedure is highly methodical involving very neat stitching, which works well for separating adhesions and not replacing them with new ones. Sometimes artificial patches are used to prevent organs sticking together again. The other advantage of this method is that there is slightly less of a risk of infection occurring afterwards.

Additional Surgical Procedures

Other operations and related tests may be performed to deal with specific problems during treatment for endometriosis. Among them are:

- Neurectomey - A surgical procedure to cut or block the nerves that transmit the pain of the disease.
- Suction evacuation - Removal with a suction device of the ovarian cysts that may accompany endometriosis
- Myomectomy - Surgical removal of fibroid growths from the uterus
- Salpingectomy - Surgical removal of a fallopian tube

- Renogram - A study of kidney function done by external monitoring radiation levels in the bladder as a radioactive chemical enters it from the kidney
- Intravenous pyelogram - an x-ray examination of the kidneys, bladder and uterus using a dye injected through a vein in the hand or arm
- Cytoscope - Examination of the wall of the bladder with a thin, lighted probe inserted through the urinary opening
- Thoracentesis - A search for endometrial blood in the lungs through a small puncture in the wall of the chest
- Proctosigmoidoscopy - Insertion of a lighted tube to search for tumours, polyps or endometrial tissue in the lower bowel
- Barium enema - An x-ray of the lower bowel to check for obstructions, deformities, tumours and polyps

Hysterectomy

The radical surgery approach is the one used on women with severe endometriosis, and usually a full hysterectomy is performed including the removal of the ovaries. It is the final major surgical approach to endometriosis. Frequently women cannot tolerate the pain and other symptoms related to endometriosis, and so they finally give in and decide on total hysterectomy. Unfortunately, these women are not aware, and probably their physicians are not aware, that endometriosis can and does come back even after hysterectomy.

Endometriosis can be found all over the abdominal cavity, and in some case in far reaching areas of the body like the lungs and the brain. So there is no point in removing the reproductive organs in the hope of removing this disease. The aim of removing the ovaries along with the uterus is to get rid of estrogen production from the body, as it is the estrogen that 'feeds' the disease. But it is not only the ovaries that produce estrogen. It is produced in smaller amounts in other areas of the body. The body will also absorb estrogen from other outside sources like the phytoestrogens found in certain foods as well as the more damaging estrogens that enter the body from chemicals in foods and chemicals used in most toiletries, which react on the body and behave like estrogen.

Women, who have had a hysterectomy, then go on to be given hormone replacement therapy, which includes of all things estrogen. HRT does include progesterone to help counter-balance the estrogen. But neither of these synthetic hormones act the same way as the ones produced by the body. The balance will be incorrect for the body to assimilate and can cause nasty side effects. Because of the renewed intake of estrogens in the body with HRT, this can then cause …. yes, **Endometriosis** to flare up again.

'I had endometriosis for 12 years during which time I had 3 laparoscopies and different types of drug treatment to try and stop the pain. With each drug treatment I would feel less pain, but the side effects were awful. After stopping the drug treatment the endo came back again. The painkillers I was trying hardly had any effect on my pain. I could not stand it any more. I eventually decided to have a hysterectomy, as I could not tolerate the pain any more. I had not had any children and I was devastated of ruining any chances of having children. But I could see no alternative to my miserable existence. After my hysterectomy I did feel better for a few months once I had recovered from the operation, but later on the pain started to come back again. I simply could not believe it. The doctors never told me that this disease could come back again even after the distress and trauma I would go through by having a hysterectomy.'

What to Ask Before any Operation

It is important to ask your consultant exactly what sort of operation you are undergoing, and to have everything explained which you do not understand. You also need to ask the following:

- How long will the operation last?
- How long will you be staying in hospital, and how long does it take to recover?
- What action will be taken if complications occur i.e. if a laparoscopy cannot help will a Laparotomy be performed?
- What symptoms can you expect after the operation?
- Is the surgeon fully trained in laparoscopic techniques?
- What type of surgical equipment/lasers do they have to be able to back up their surgical needs?
- What will you feel as soon as your come round from the operation - getting an answer to this one really helps alleviate the fear and anxiety many people suffer when they wake from surgery
- What sort of stitches will you have - will they be dissolvable or have to be removed later
- How should you look after yourself when you go home i.e. how to move the body, any gentle exercise to aid recovery

What to Ask after the Operation

When you have recovered from your operation, it is important to ask the surgeon exactly what has been done. This is often done at a follow-up appointment, if not done at the time of the procedure. Women are often given insufficient information about their problem. You should consider asking the following questions:

- What degree of endometriosis was found?
- How extensive was it?
- Which organs were affected?
- Were there any adhesions?
- Were your bowel or reproductive organs affected in any way?
- How many cysts were found and how large were they?
- How successful was the treatment at removing the endometriosis?
- Were any adhesions repaired?
- Are your fallopian tubes clear?
- Did the operation go well? i.e. were there any minor complications?
- What are your future prospects for conception and having children?

You will no doubt have other questions of your own; so write down a list to take to the hospital with you. Make sure the list is kept safe while you have your operation. It may be no good returning to your surgeon a few weeks or months after the operation to get advice, as he or she may not remember your case so well.

Laparoscopy Advice

For most women going into hospital for the first time to have a Laparoscopy can be a worrying time. The emotional anxiety about what the surgeon will find will cause as much concern as the actual process of having an operation. I have put together here a list of tips, ideas and advice to help you get prepared for your laparoscopy.

Preparation

If you are well prepared the whole experience will be less traumatic and frightening. It is also vital to obtain information from your consultant or gynaecologist as to what they intend to achieve during your laparoscopy. If you are unclear of anything they say, ask for a better explanation. You will no doubt have many questions and concerns. Write these down and discuss them in your pre-op appointment with your consultant.

You will want to know what surgical options there are for the treatment of endometriosis. This will depend on the training and experience of your particular consultant. You will also want to know how your consultant can deal with different stages of the disease. Each laparoscopy will be different as no two women are the same, and there are no set patterns to this disease.

If you are member of an endometriosis support group in your area, talk to other women in the group of their experiences and what they did that helped when they had a laparoscopy.

Prepare Practicalities

There are many small but very useful things you can do to make the whole process of undergoing surgery and recovery much easier. Much of this is about preparing things around the home and in your life so that you can focus on resting and recovery when you get back home.

- Prepare your food stocks so that you have all the provisions you will need. If you live with a partner then they will be doing the cooking, but if you live alone you need to buy in some frozen or instant meals. Better still, cook and freeze your own meals in advance. I personally find convenience ready meals full of nasty additives and preservatives that I do not want in my body. This is even more relevant when I need extra support from my food intake to help me heal and look after my body.
- Clean your home the day before surgery, then you come home to a nice environment
- Change the linen on your bed the day before surgery, again for the pleasure of nice clean sheets, and you will not be capable for changing the linen for at least a week by yourself
- Make sure you have a supply of sanitary towels, pain killers, hot water bottle, buy some magazines to read at leisure, rent or borrow some videos to entertain you
- Make sure you have 2 or 3 loose fitting outfits. You will not want to be wearing anything tight, especially round the abdomen
- Start taking extra Vitamin C for about 2 weeks prior to the operation - this will help your body deal with the anaesthetic as well as help with healing
- Purchase Homeopathic Remedies - Arnica 30c - you will use this to assist healing and relieve pain after surgery. Phosphorus 6c - to relieve vomiting after anaesthetic
- Purchase some throat lozenges - to help with the sore throat caused by the tube which is put down your throat during the operation
- Inform friends and family of your operation date and the time you expect to be back home. This will allow them the opportunity to keep in touch and see how you are. Also put your phone by the bed for easy reach.
- Obviously if you have children you will have to make child care arrangements. If you have pets, especially a dog, you need to make arrangements for dog walking

Prepare Yourself

- The day before - eat light and healthy and drink lots of fluids. Do not eat or drink anything after 12.00 midnight the night before surgery. Do not smoke or chew gum after 12.00 midnight If your surgery is scheduled for later in the day, it is advised to have some supper around 11.00pm so you are not totally starving throughout the next day
- Your doctor or consultant will probably ask you to do an enema in the evening to clean out your bowel. If more severe endometriosis is suspected, then a full bowel prep may be required. You will be given instructions on this during your pre-op office visit. Preparing the bowel with a purging agent such as Magnesium Citrate is often followed by an oral antibiotic and enemas. While unpleasant, this procedure minimises the risk of surgical complications from bowel injury during surgery.
- Pack a hospital bag including: warm, loose clothing to wear after the operation, wash-kit, phone book - should you need to contact someone, sanitary towels, a blank video - if you are having your procedure taped, something to read if you have to wait around for your turn in theatre, clean socks to keep your feet warm during surgery. Leave your wallet and valuables at home.
- Remove all nail polish, remove jewellery and contact lenses
- Ensure that you have a lift home from hospital. If this has been prearranged with a friend some time beforehand, ring them a few days before to ensure they remember.
- Take a long warm bath the night before, drink some camomile tea to aid restful sleep, and get a good nights sleep.

The Day of Surgery

- Try to get up early, take a shower if you wish and put on comfortable clothing. Do not bother doing much to your hair; it will only be put into a protective cap for the operation. Do not forget that you are not allowed breakfast. Do not wear any make-up, perfume, hair spray or deodorant.
- Arrive at the hospital at the designated time to register. There will be forms to fill in and consent forms to sign. Ensure that you specify what you do NOT want to have done during surgery.
- The process of signing in to hospital on the day of your treatment will vary for different countries, but the actual medical procedure will be similar. You will probably be shown to your bed and given instructions by a member of the ward staff. This usually involves instructions for getting undressed and changed into hospital gowns, putting any belongings into safe keeping, and then advised to wait for consultations with the medical staff. You will get a visit from your consultant and one from the anaesthesiologist.
- You need to discuss with the anaesthesiologist any fears or worries you have. They will ask you about any allergies you may have or whether there is any family history of bad reaction to anaesthesia.
- Depending which country you are having treatment, you will probably be given a pre-op shot which makes you feel very drowsy and floaty. This helps to alleviate some of the nervousness. This is usually given about an hour before the operation.
- When it is time to go to theatre for your surgery, you will be collected. In the UK this is done by porters who put you on a trolley, cover you in blankets to keep you warm and you are wheeled off down endless corridors in a drowsy state.

- You will arrive at the theatre suite, in a prep room just outside of theatre. The anaesthesiologist will make sure you are ready and will then insert an IV (intra-venous) needle into the back of your hand. A tube is then fitted to the IV ready for the anaesthetic to flow directly into your system. The anaesthesiologist will ask you to start counting backwards from 100, keeping your eyes open. You will feel a cold rush into the back of your hand as the anaesthetic starts to flow into your system. Most people do not get much further than counting down to about 80.

Surgical Recovery

You will not remember anything else until after your operation. Depending on which country you live in, you will either come round from the surgery in the recovery room or you will back on the ward in your bed.

You will be feeling very groggy and unsure of where you are at first. You will then begin to focus your thoughts for a while and will realise that you are back safe in the real world again. You will drift in and out of sleep for a few hours whilst the anaesthetic wears off. A nurse should come and take your temperature and check your pulse and blood pressure at regular intervals.

As you begin to come round a bit more you will start to feel the different pains in your body. You will have pain where the incisions were made; your abdomen will feel sore and painful from the operation as well as being distended by the gas. The worse pain noted by most women is a sharp stabbing pain in the shoulder. This is a side effect of the gas that is used to distend the abdomen, which seems to travel around the system. The pain can feel as though a sword has been driven through you. So watch out for this one.

You need to ask for painkillers if you suffering a lot. You can also be given something to help with the nausea. You need to try sipping some water if you feel up to it. Many people feel too nauseous to let anything pass their lips.

This is a good time to take some Phosphorus - the Homeopathic remedy - to help you stop feeling so queasy. Take one dose every half hour until you start to feel more settled. You can then start to get some fluid into your system and drink some water. You also need to start taking some Arnica - the other Homeopathic remedy - to help speed up recovery and reduce the pain.

You will find yourself continuing to drift in and out of sleep very easily for a few more hours. Do try to get up at some point and go to the toilet to urinate. This will sting because of the catheter that is inserted for the operation. If you are having treatment on a day-care basis you will not be allowed to go home until you have urinated. This is to ensure that your system is working correctly.

If you staying at the hospital overnight then you will be given something very light to eat before the day is over. This will help to level out your blood-sugar levels and will improve how you feel.

Your first night will be rather uncomfortable with abdominal pain, feeling groggy from the operation, and an awful shifting pain in your shoulders, which hurts every time you move around. The pain is at its worse when you try to sit up. Do your best to lie still for your first night, and try not to get to distressed about the results of your surgery.

You may have been given your results on the day of the operation but in most cases your consultant will inform you of the outcome the following day if you are staying overnight.

If you are a day-case, you can go home once you feel ready for the journey and the medical staff are happy with your vital signs. Those who are staying over-night will be checked over in the morning and will probably go home around mid-morning.

For your journey home, ensure someone is going to collect you. You will NOT be able to drive yourself. It is a good idea to have a small cushion to hold against your abdomen. This helps to protect you from sudden bumps in the road. It is also advisable and more comfortable to recline your seat slightly.

Get out of the car carefully AND GO TO BED.

Recovery at Home

For the first few days you need to stay in bed and get as much sleep as possible. You will have bleeding which will be similar to having a period, which is normal.

- The incision near the navel can be rather sore. If you have had another incision lower on the abdomen this will also need protecting. Do not wear any clothing that is going to rub on these incisions. Follow your doctors instructions on cleaning and dressing the incisions and watch for signs of infection.
- The stitches used in the incisions are usually the type that dissolve so you do not need to return to hospital to have them removed
- It can take a few days for the shoulder pains caused by the gas to finally stop. It will also make you belch a lot.
- Your abdomen will be bloated for a few days, but will gradually go down
- The amount of surgical pain and cramping you have depends on how extensive your surgery was. Use painkillers and a hot water bottle or heating pad.
- Just take things steady for the first few days. Try to get up and walk around the house a little bit. You may feel dizzy and weak, but it is better that lying in bed and not moving at all, which will make you feel worse when you do try to get up.
- Your diet needs to be very light and simple for the first few days. You may find that you are constipated which is caused by a combination of the anaesthetic, lack of bodily movement, lack of food intake, and the effects of painkillers.
- Drink lots of fluids, especially pure water, fruit juices, herb teas. Increase you bulk intake after 2 days. It is best not to eat too much at first. Digestion taxes the system and requires energy for digestion to take place. It is best to reserve this energy for healing and let your body get over the shock.
- Gradually get back into normal routine over a period of about a week, increasing what you do every day.
- Do not try to bend over to pick things up - it hurts far too much. Bend at the knees instead and drop your weight down to pick things up.
- Continue taking a few doses of Arnica each day to help speed your recover

Returning to Daily Life

Your healing will be steady and gradual over the period of about 2 weeks before you start to feel somewhat normal again. I would not personally advise going back to work for a least a week, and this is only if you do a desk job. If you do any physical work - which most women with endometriosis cannot anyway - but you need to consider having at least 3 weeks off work

* * *

A Final Word about Laparoscopy surgery

A laparoscopy in itself is not a major operation - the basic procedure is to allow visual inspection of the abdomen and entails a small incision in the abdomen and a viewing instrument is inserted. A laparoscopy becomes a major surgery when treatment is included and your surgeon then uses other instruments to deal with the endometriosis. This can include cutting or burning away cysts, cutting or burning adhesions, and treating any other complications caused by endometriosis.

It is when the latter is extensive that having a laparoscopy is a major operation and recovery time will take longer. Do not rush your recovery, allow the body to heal itself gradually and you will reap the rewards of being able to return to daily life without any setbacks.

Final Thoughts regarding Treatment

It is extremely important that women with endometriosis seek to obtain their treatment from a highly trained endometriosis specialist if they can. There are many inexperienced physicians out there who can get it wrong. This may involve:

- missing the disease altogether and not perform tissue biopsies to confirm the diagnosis
- will confirm the disease but make no attempt to remove it during surgery
- will not remove the disease properly during operation
- not providing unbiased treatment options

When considering your treatment options you need to think about the following:

- All surgical procedures carry the element of risk
- All drug therapy is going to have side-effects
- It is not known how long lasting the side-effects from drugs can be
- Having an anaesthetic can stay in your system for months
- Find out all you can about each treatment being offered, so you can be prepared, for example, you can prepare your body for an operation by good nutrition
- If you intend to start, or maintain your treatment using modern drug and chemical therapy, then do as much as you can to look after your body, to give it support.
- Get as much help as you can from friends and family. If they do not understand this disease then lend them this book, lend them some leaflets, a magazine article, anything, so they understand.
- You will need lots of help and support especially after an operation, or if you are trying to adjust to new drug treatment.
- Be kind to yourself, do not push yourself too hard.

Other Health Problems Related to Endometriosis

It is rather poignant to including this section, as the subject matter just seems to add more doom and gloom. Many of you may be aware of the research and findings about other health problems in women with endometriosis.

From what I have been reading, it appears that women with endometriosis are much more likely to suffer from other serious health problems. I want to emphasise the word likely because these findings do not mean you will definitely have, or definitely develop these other health problems.

There are other symptoms with endometriosis which most women, including myself have had to deal with (like the bowel problems, insomnia, low grade infections etc). These symptoms seem to relate directly to the diseased state of endometriosis. But these other serious health issues we are starting to hear about are not directly related, they are separate diseases. This seems to indicate, or should I say strengthen the case that endometriosis is another immune system deficiency.

Here are some of the findings from data collected from the world's largest research registry on endometriosis.

- Women with endometriosis and their families have a heightened risk of breast cancer, melanoma and ovarian cancer
- Chronic fatigue syndrome is more than 100 times more common in women with endometriosis
- There is a high rate of thyroid disorders in women with endometriosis, as well as their families. Hypothyroidism, which involves an under active thyroid and causes mental and physical slowing, is seven times more common
- Other autoimmune diseases which are seen significantly in women with endometriosis and their families, include Rheumatoid Arthritis, Lupus, Multiple Sclerosis, Meniere's disease
- Fibromyalgia, which is characterised by widespread body pain and tiredness, is twice as common
- Allergic conditions are much higher, occurring in approximately 60 percent of women with endometriosis

I have a few thoughts coming from these findings.

Why is it that these other diseases are also becoming more common in the families of women with endometriosis? None of these diseases or disorders can be caught, and then passed onto another member of the family. So are these statistics related to geographic location, where the environment these women and their families are living is much more toxic, and having an effect on the immune system of the entire family. This situation seems somewhat plausible to me. It has been cited that the risk of endometriosis is increased when there is a genetic autoimmune dysfunction in the family. This could explain the 'rash' of illnesses within one family.

In the past endometriosis has been viewed in isolation, as a singular diseased state of the individual, and not been put into context to include the other health problems women face with this disease. It has not been put into context of the environment where these women live. It has not been viewed to include the health issues of her family. But now this is finally being done, a bigger and more complex picture is beginning to emerge.

Looking at some of the other health crises, and diseases that are cropping up, it almost looks as though the disease of endometriosis is acting as a warning flag and providing strong signals that the health of the general populace is at risk as well. We only have to look at the statistics of the number of increasing cases of endometriosis, and the fact that it is rising sharply in the industrialised world.

What is the Cause of Endometriosis?

This is the million-dollar question. No one knows what causes endometriosis. No fewer than 12 theories have been proposed since 1921 to explain how and why this disease occurs. John Sampson, MD first developed the reflux menstruation theory in 1920.

These are some of the common theories of the cause, or trigger for endometriosis

- Retrograde or reflux menstruation - Dr Sampson believed that during a woman's period some menstrual fluid flowed backwards from the uterus to 'shower the pelvic organs and pelvis lining' with endometrial cells
- The transplant theory - endometriosis spreads via the circulatory and lymphatic system
- Hereditary - women whose close relatives have the disease are at higher risk of developing it
- Iatrogenic transplantation - endometriosis is accidentally transported during abdominal surgery
- Coelomic metaplasia - certain cells, when stimulated, can transform themselves into a different kind of cell, as in women taking estrogen-replacement therapy, and in men, who following prostate removal, have received estrogen
- Immunology - endometriosis develops in certain women who are deficient in certain immune cells
- Environmental chemicals - A great deal of research has been done to suggest that chemical toxins in the environment are the root cause of endometriosis, because when they enter the body they mimic certain hormones

There are certain factors that have been cited to increase the risk of endometriosis which include:

- estrogen excess
- progesterone deficiency
- magnesium deficiency
- essential fatty acid deficiency
- high fat diet, especially animal fats
- high stress load
- hormone imbalance
- excess dietary caffeine
- excess alcohol

The broader issues, ideas, and speculations of the possible cause or causes of endometriosis are covered in part three. There we go into more detail, referring to a broader range of topics on this subject. Being made aware of these issues will inform you of the gravity and seriousness of just how many things can be affecting your health and possibly why you may have developed endometriosis.

How Endometriosis Affects your Life

The way endometriosis affects your life is very often over-looked by people who are not directly affected by this disease. Endometriosis affects a woman's life far beyond the physical symptoms of the disease. If you have been suffering from endometriosis for some time, then you will know exactly what I mean. For those of you who have just been diagnosed, or those women who suspect that they may have endometriosis, then it is best that you begin to understand, that your life will change.

I personally found out gradually, the total impact that endometriosis was to have on my life, as I said in my story. Then, the further the disease progressed, the harder the truth hit home. I am not saying this to be negative, or to scare you, but I feel it is best to be honest, and for you to be prepared. I was not prepared, and it was frightening, I felt lonely and it was hell. There simply was not the same amount of information and support available as there is today.

Endometriosis and Relationships

The way endometriosis affects your relationships can be very obvious but it can also be very, very subtle. The most profound affect it can have is on your relationship with your partner if you have one. Even if you do not have a partner, it affects your image of yourself and how you imagine not being able to sustain a loving relationship whilst dealing with the symptoms of endometriosis.

Partners

The repercussions of endometriosis on you and your partner are constant. It is something that is there day in, day out. You will probably be suffering from constant tiredness, which can make every day tasks seem like a huge effort. The tiredness will make you more miserable and depressed than you already are. It becomes a vicious circle.

You will have the depression to deal with because of the pain and you are also aware of the possible long-term affects of endometriosis regarding fertility and starting a family, if you have not got children already. Both you and your partner will no doubt go through agonies over this.

There will be so many things in life that you will not be able to do now due to lack of energy or the pain of endometriosis, which could be constant or it could be at certain times of the month.

This disease can be one of the most testing and trying situations for a close relationship. I do know that some marriages and long-term relationships have been ruined because of endometriosis. This situation is so sad, but in a long-term relationship where both partners want a family and that situation looks to be in jeopardy, then sometimes the strain is just too much. Added to this is the difficulty of having a normal, healthy sex life because of the pain it can cause. The affect of this goes to the core of a relationship, and sometimes it can be too much to deal with, and can also cause the break up of a relationship.

There are many women however, who find themselves in a relationship with a man who is in it for real, in sickness and in health, and they do as much as they can to provide support and help cope with the broader concerns that this disease brings up. There are now support groups springing up on the Internet, dedicated to provide support for men whose partners have endometriosis. This will help to alleviate the isolation for these men and give them a network where they can share experiences.

There are no easy answers as to how to improve the quality of your relationship with your partner when you are trying to cope with a serious illness. It all comes down to the qualities, the attitudes, the personalities, the needs, and so many other personal traits of the individuals involved.

It has been found by other women suffering from endometriosis, that when they educate their partners and their family about endometriosis, they then begin to understand just what a profound affect this disease is having on the woman and her image of herself. The more they learn, the more they understand, and the closer they feel, which has improved their relationships immensely.

Friends

Your relationships with your friends will undoubtedly change, sometimes for the worse, and this can be very hurtful. This will not be intentional and there will be no malice, it just happens. It seems to go with the territory of illness. They will be concerned at first; they will offer support and advice. They will visit you in hospital when you have yet another operation. But gradually this support starts to wear thin. Your friends still want you to be the person they knew before. The person who could go out for the evening at a moments notice. The person who was full of energy and enjoyed a good laugh.

Now, you have to plan everything around your periods. You feel too awful to even leave your bed most months. And you dread it, if for any reason your periods go haywire and do not start on time. This can happen, and you may be out for the evening and suddenly you start having serious agonising cramps. You just have to put your coat on, tell the friend you were sat next to that you feel bad and have to go home. You walk away from your crowd of friends, who are all laughing, joking and having a good night out with the girls. You look over your shoulder, you feel gutted, and none of your friends realise just how bad you feel. It is an awful, lonely, lonely feeling. I know, I have been there. The people you used to share so much with are now fading into the background.

You may be lucky to have a few friends who are more sensitive and understanding, and they will continue to be good friends no matter how awful you are feeling. These are the sort of people who can visualise how they would like to be treated if it was they who were ill. But the strange thing that happens to most people regarding illness is they have an innate tendency to shy away from other people who are ill. They do not want to associate with it, to face up to it, and to realise that "it could happen to anyone of us". ….. It is the understanding souls who will stay in contact. The ones who have a true sense of reality including all of life's pitfalls.

Co-workers

What happens with your work colleagues is very similar as to what happens with your friends, and they gradually draw away. They do not want to get involved in your 'tales of woe'.

But the serious affect it has is on your career credibility. You will probably end up taking time off work because you are not fit enough to work. You will have the same nightmarish attitudes to deal with here as you do with your doctor, in that they cannot see anything physically wrong with you, so it must be one of those typical 'women things' that is bothering you.

Many women will continue to try and work when they do not feel well enough, but they will be performing below par. Your manager/boss will notice this; they will ask if anything is wrong, you try to explain in a brief succinct manner, but the gravity of your situation 'does not compute'! You may as well be talking to a brick wall.

It gets to the point were you dread going to work, because of the things that are being said behind your back. People do not like it when colleagues are off sick because they have to fill in for them. They also feel resentment based on selfish human nature. They too would like to go into work when it suits them and not to have to continually work the contracted 5 days a week, every week. So they feel you are only going into work when it suits you, not knowing that you are off sick for a genuine reason. And so the animosity builds, and when you get back to work the atmosphere is awful.

Eventually, you end up in a situation where your work quality and sickness leave puts you in a situation were you are given a warning about your conduct in your job. This happened to me and it just added another insult to injury.

You then start to look for work that is part time or even to stop work all together if you can manage financially. All this has come about due to inconsiderate and uncaring attitudes in the work place. This leads me onto my next subject where endometriosis affects your life.

Endometriosis and Economic Factors

The financial cost of coping with endometriosis is far-reaching and can be crippling in itself.

Firstly, as I have just mentioned it can have an enormous affect on your income earning potential, as you may have difficulty in holding onto your job, or not even capable of working at all.

If that is the case then you should be claiming for Disability Benefit (or whatever it is called in your country). It is now beginning to be recognised by the welfare state in different countries that endometriosis is a **disabling disease** and as such is eligible for a claim for Disability Benefit. But it is not always that easy to claim. You may need to go to an independent doctor for an assessment of your incapacity to work. Sometimes these doctors can be very dismissive, and usually do not understand how serious endometriosis is. We are back to the problem of lack of knowledge of the disease.

If you find yourself having to go for an assessment, then take as much printed information about the disease that can validate the fact that what you are dealing with is a serious, painful, debilitating disease. Print off information from the Internet that comes from informed sources. Get onto the Internet to find out your rights regarding your claim for benefit. Get the up to date information, as this legislation changes so often. Find out if you can claim, even if you are living with a partner. There are different rules for different countries, so I cannot go into this in detail here.

Treatment costs

On top of the financial stress of how to have enough money to live on each week, especially if you are single, there is the cost of treatment. This is of primary concern to women who live in the US who are not privy to a National Health Service.

The cost of paying for treatment can seriously mount up if you have to pay for your treatment either because there is no free health care service or you decide to go private. The figures quoted here are relevant for the US, which will vary from one part of the country to another.

At the time of writing the average cost of a Laparoscopy is between $4,000 to $6,000, depending on the extent of the disease. This does not include the hospital charges. This figure is purely for the cost of the actual operation.

A Laparotomy will cost between $6,000 to $7,000 plus the hospital costs

Treatment with hormone medications (usually 6 to 9 months) costs between $225 to $350 PER MONTH. This does not include the cost of monitoring tests and physician charges. So if a woman is on drug treatment for 6 months and is paying an average of $300 per month for the drugs, plus the doctor's charges, plus the tests, this could come to well over $3,000.

There will be many women who simply cannot afford this amount of money, so they cannot afford their treatment. This situation is diabolical when you consider the HUGE profits that are being made by drug and pharmaceutical companies all over the world.

Many women are also using a variety of dietary supplements, vitamins, herbs and alternative treatments, all of which adds up in cost. Some women are doing a lot to improve their diet, and many of them aim to go organic as much as possible. Organic food is more expensive than produce provided in mainstream supermarkets. The main reason to go organic is to try and cut out the pesticides and pollutants, all of which aggravate endometriosis. There is more on this subject later.

The financial burden of endometriosis on a day-to-day basis, without the cost of the actual treatment, is one that is hard to cope with for women of limited income. The situation regarding Disability Benefit is improving, and if you include as much authoritative information about endometriosis in support of your claim, then you should have success. If you do not, THEN APPEAL. If you need support or help go to your Citizens Advice Bureau (for UK residents) or similar advice office. Find out if there are other women in a support group who live near you, who have any literature or up to date information to help with your claim for Disability Benefit.

Sense of Identity

The affects of endometriosis on a woman's identity and self-esteem are immense. Her image of herself will become distorted because endometriosis hits at the root of her femininity.

A woman may feel out of control and may worry about her worth as a partner. Firstly there is the heart-breaking issue of not being able to enjoy a happy and healthy sex life. Then there is the fear, guilt, anger and worry that she may not be able to conceive.

There is the constant worry if a woman is in a relationship that her partner may leave her because, in her mind, she feels she is not sexually desirable, may not be able to have children and is generally not fit and well. For a woman who is still single and wishes to settle down, she may wonder how on earth she tells her prospective partner that she may have difficulty having children.

The affects of some of the drug treatment can have awful side effects on a woman's psyche, as well as physical side effects. As I mentioned earlier, they can cause depression, weight-gain, and loss of libido, to name but a few. There is the added worry regarding long-term risks of taking the drug treatment, like the risk of heart disease and osteoporosis.

Trying to deal with the pain, which for many women seems to be on a daily basis, and can be relentless, can cause further depression and tiredness.

Then you add to that the financial burden, the difficulty of holding down a job, not being able to sustain your friendships, not being able to have an active social life, and generally feeling as though life is closing down. A feeling that all life is about is endometriosis.

These are all huge psychological stresses that are faced by most women with endometriosis, and it has a huge impact on a woman and her family. Many women will feel very isolated and alone in their ordeal. This is why women must seek help, find support from other women who have endometriosis, and get themselves and their families and loved ones educated about this disease. Gaining knowledge is the first step towards taking control.

Endometriosis and Infertility

For countless women one of the most devastating consequences of endometriosis is possible infertility and the overall effect is has on her fertility. Not only does she have to deal with a debilitating disease and all the pain it brings, she may also have to deal with loosing her chances of motherhood and being infertile. This simply adds insult to injury for those women who were keen to have children of their own.

But let's not paint a totally gloomy picture here. It is fortunate that not all women who have endometriosis are infertile. It is estimated that around 40 percent of women with endometriosis are infertile. If all women with endometriosis were infertile then birth rates would drop considerably and a rush to find successful treatment for this disease would, hopefully, be implemented.

It has been found that between 30 to 40 percent of women undergoing laparoscopy as part of an infertility evaluation are found to have endometriosis. This is when women are finally diagnosed with the disease by default.

There appear to be a number of mechanisms by which endometriosis impacts on fertility. Scarring or adhesions in the pelvis, for example, can cause much infertility. The fallopian tubes and ovaries may adhere to the lining of the pelvis or to each other, restricting their movement. The scarring and adhesions that takes place with endometriosis may mean that the ovaries and fallopian tubes are not in the right position, so the transfer of the egg to the fallopian tubes cannot take place. Similarly, endometriosis can cause damage and/or blockage to the inside of the fallopian tube, impeding the journey of the egg down the fallopian tube to the uterus.

Another factor, which could cause infertility for women with endometriosis, may be the over-production of prostaglandins. These are hormones that play an important role in the fertilisation and implantation of the embryo. An excess of prostaglandins may interfere with these processes.

Because endometriosis often causes painful intercourse, couples may fail to have intercourse during the woman's most fertile time, which will obviously impede the possibility of conception.

Not only does endometriosis affect a woman's overall fertility and her ability to become pregnant, it also affects her ability to remain pregnant. Several studies have indicated that women with untreated endometriosis have a spontaneous abortion rate of approximately 40 to 50 percent, in contrast to the 10 to 15 percent abortion rate in the general population.

Statistically women with endometriosis have fewer children than women who do not have the disease. When looking at the medical history of women before their endometriosis is diagnosed, many of them are much more likely to have had not only spontaneous abortion, but also tubal pregnancies, premature labours and stillborn babies.

The stage or extent of the disease does not indicate the infertility of a woman who has endometriosis. It is true that higher stages (3 and 4) are more likely to be infertile, but not always strictly the case.

A Closer Look at some of the Causes of Infertility

Abdominal Adhesions and Infertility

As the endometriosis implants grow and develop in the abdomen, the body tries to surround them with fibrous connective tissue (scar tissue). The body does this in an attempt to isolate the implants and prevent them from doing harm. Adhesions can also be formed during surgery when abdominal tissue is traumatised.

These fibrous growths also have the affect of making the implants stick to adjacent tissue, and in some case organs can be 'glued' together. Also the blood from internal bleeding from the implants can forms adhesions, so that an implant may be stuck to several different tissues. For example, an endometriosis implant on the top of the uterus may cause the ovary and small intestine to become attached at the site of the implant.

If the adhesions caused by endometriosis pinch off the fallopian tube or if they cause blockage to the opening of the fallopian tube, they could obstruct the merger of egg and sperm and prevent fertilisation and conception. Also ectopic pregnancy is more common with endometriosis, if the embryo can't travel to the womb. This type of obstruction can be easily diagnosed and surgically corrected.

However, this does not explain how patients with just a few endometriosis implants and no adhesions can become infertile. Adhesions can also cause pain, as internal organs which normally slip and slide are firmly glued together. For example, if the bowel is stuck to a tender, painful ovary, flatulence could cause pain.

Secretions from implants

The normal endometrium which lines the womb is a very active and vital tissue that secretes a wide variety of nutrients and hormones required for normal conception. The endometriosis implants also secrete these same substances, but instead of depositing them into the lumen (centre) of the womb as normal, the endometriosis implants release their chemical secretions into the abdominal cavity. Some of these substances are potent hormones which could interfere with fertility.

Prostaglandins

One major group of hormones secreted by the normal endometrium is that of the prostaglandins. Prostaglandins are oil-based hormones found in nearly all the tissues of the body and are required for many bodily processes, including several stages of the menstrual cycle and pregnancy.

Prostaglandins are required for ovulation, regression of the corpus luteum (i.e., ending the monthly menstrual cycle), sperm motility, immune interaction, contraction of the uterus at birth and menstrual cramps. Endometriosis implants and the endometrium of the uterus are the richest source of prostaglandin production in the body.

However, the problem with endometriosis implants include:
  - Prostaglandins are released into the abdomen instead of inside the womb
  - Prostaglandins release by the implants seem to be out of phase with their release by the
    uterus.
  - Prostaglandins are produced at the wrong time sending the wrong message.

For instance, there is a normal surge in prostaglandin F production at the end of the menstrual cycle, causing the effect of the corpus luteum of the ovary to die down and signalling the start of a new menstrual cycle. The implants of endometriosis produce their own prostaglandin surge several days after that of the womb lining. This may be one of the main causes of very early miscarriage.

If a women is a few days pregnant then the endometriosis implants producing prostaglandin F would incorrectly signal the ovary to start a new menstrual cycle, causing the womb lining with the implanted egg to be expelled - and the consequence is an early miscarriage.

Prostaglandins also play an important role in the contractions of womb and fallopian tubes. During the normal menstrual cycle, the gentle contraction of the womb and fallopian tube aids the movement of egg and sperm to the outer third of the fallopian tube where fertilisation occurs. High concentrations of endometriosis implants may prevent fertilisation. An excess of PGF2 and PGE2 could cause contractions that are too strong and expel the egg too quickly.

Early Miscarriage

The most common time for a miscarriage to occur is during the first three months of pregnancy. During this time, the embryo is developing into a foetus and is undergoing dramatic changes, including the formation of most of its internal organs. This is a critical period of development that requires an appropriate nutrient-rich environment, a healthy placenta and a very delicate balance between the various hormones of pregnancy.

However, the real problem of a an early miscarriage, is that if it occurs during the first six weeks of pregnancy, there is a good chance that women may not even be aware that they were pregnant. They may simply think their period was late.

Regardless of whether or not there is a high miscarriage rate in endometriosis patients, it is imperative to eat the right sort of nutrient-rich food to try to ensure the maintenance of a pregnancy. Nutrition in both parents, even before pregnancy has a profound effect on the state of the egg and sperm, as well as on the nature of the secretions within the peritoneal cavity. Choice of foods, particularly fats and oils, may be a crucial factor as these affect the production of prostaglandins, cell membranes, steroid hormones, and neurotransmitters etc.

Fertility and the Alert Immune System

In order to achieve pregnancy, sperm has to enter the body. This sperm can be judged as 'alien' by a woman's immune cells, because it is 'non-self'. If pregnancy is achieved, the women's immune system has to adapt to the presence of 'alien' tissue growing inside her for nine months.

However, there will be some mechanism in nature, which tells the female immune system that this alien tissue is not a danger, in order to avoid damage to the embryo. Perhaps when the immune system is malfunctioning in endometriosis, this mechanism fails and causes an immune attack on the embryo and sperm, thought to lead to infertility. Correcting or strengthening the immune system may help to achieve fertility for women with endometriosis

Fertility Treatment

Nearly every woman who has endometriosis will be worried about the condition of her fertility and her ability to have children. Motherhood is such a fundamental focus and role for most women, even for women who have rewarding and demanding careers.

After treatment for endometriosis some women go on to have further treatment to assist with successful conception. There are also a few measures you can take to help yourself and aid successful conception.

Your most Fertile Time

Some people are not aware that there is a relatively short time each month when a woman can get pregnant. The key time for peak fertility is 48 hours after the egg is released. But in total there is a period of approximately 7 days when you can conceive, because the sperm can survive for about five days inside the woman's body awaiting for the egg. So five days before the egg is released (which is usually Day 14 of a 28 day cycle) and two days after are your most fertile times. Buying an ovulation prediction kit, which measures the hormones in your urine, may help you to know your peak fertile time.

Temperature Charts

A simple and inexpensive aid to infertility treatment is keeping a temperature chart, which measures your basal body temperature (BBT). There is a change in the BBT which relate to the monthly cycle of ovulation. This temperature is charted by taking your measuring your body temperature first thing in the morning before rising. There are special BBT thermometers available for this purpose.

By plotting the changes in temperature a woman can identify her most fertile time of the month which can be especially useful for women who suffer from pain with intercourse, so that they can time intercourse appropriately and avoid painful sexual activity during less fertile times.

Infertility Tests

Blood tests: These are usually done on Day 21 of your cycle. The test is done to show the levels of the various reproductive hormones in your bloodstream. Your partner may also take a semen test for analysis at the same time.

Post-coital tests: If the blood and semen tests prove inconclusive, you may have a post-coital test whereby mucus from the cervix is sent for analysis after sex. If live, active sperm are seen, then the tests are normal.

If there are problems with either of these, further tests may follow.

X-ray: An HSG (hysterosalpingogram, an x-ray of the uterus and fallopian tubes) is often used to determine the health of the reproductive organs, as part of infertility evaluation. This test will show whether the tubes are open and may reveal abnormalities of the uterus. A Laparoscopy may be advised to determine the extent of damage to the organs and surgical repair can take place where possible.

IVF

IVF stands for in vitro fertilisation. It is normally used in conjunction with a fertility drug like Clomid. Recent research, which is still in the investigative phase, may indicate that the fertility drug Clomid might cause extra implantation problems in the lining of the uterus of a woman who has endometriosis.

This drug is also used for fertility treatment. It is used to treat ovulation failure, and works by stimulating the ovaries into producing several mature eggs at one time. This is why it is so common for women to have multiple births when they have received fertility treatment.

During IVF the woman is monitored with ultrasound equipment to find out when one of the ovary sacs will burst open. As the time approaches, a fine needle is passed through the wall of the abdomen to suck out some of the ripe eggs, which are then mixed with the partner's sperm. Once fertilisation has taken place, the eggs are put directly into the womb.

GIFT

GIFT stands for Gamete Intra-Fallopian Transfer, and means that the gametes (the sperm and egg) are put back into the womb at an earlier stage than in ordinary IVF treatment. They are usually flushed into the Fallopian tubes where fertilisation may be more likely to take place because of the more natural environment.

Success with Pregnancy

Many doctors feel that for a woman who has endometriosis, the best chances of a natural pregnancy occur during the six to nine months period following treatment with a laparoscopy procedure.

There are many women with endometriosis who do succeed in having children. For some of these women these pregnancies may have taken place without treatment for endometriosis; their pregnancies would have happened anyway. There is no way of knowing. For other women, they have successfully conceived after some form of medical treatment.

Other women are achieving pregnancy without any conventional medical intervention for endometriosis, and are simply taking care of their own health though alternative treatments. This may include changes in diet or getting treatment from an alternative health practitioner. Success with pregnancy has been achieved by using Homeopathy, Acupuncture, Traditional Chinese Medicine, Herbalism, to name a few, as well as following self-help programmes including vitamins and supplements and diet changes.

For some women, their pregnancy success has come about by combining conventional treatment for endometriosis along with Complimentary therapies.

To address the problems with infertility and endometriosis and achieve successful pregnancy may require a combination of treatments. This means correcting hormone imbalances that have been directly caused by endometriosis; then to repair the structure of the reproductive organs.

This is probably best achieved by:

- natural therapies to rebalance hormones, boost the immune system and reduce active endometriosis
- changing the diet to achieve optimum health and nutrition
- followed with surgery to correct damage to the structure of the reproductive organs to allow for successful conception

Natural and Alternative therapies can work wonders to restore health and bring the body back into balance, but surgery may be needed in some cases to repair damaged tissue and organs caused by endometriosis and to restore them close to their original function. There is a more detailed explanation of the reasons for the possible need of surgery in the last chapter, from the viewpoint of using natural/alternative treatment.

* * *

Successful Pregnancy
using Traditional Chinese Medicine

'31 year old Emily presented to the clinic with a chief complaint of painful periods and trying to conceive with no luck for five years. She was accompanied by her husband, and appeared very shaky and upset. She had had a diagnosis of endometriosis from her gynaecologist. She had two surgeries; a D&C with myomectomy, and laparoscopy to remove adhesions on her ovaries and uterus 13 months after the first operation. She had just completed her third intrauterine insemination attempt after twelve cycles of Clomid, all of which failed. She stated that she was very sensitive to the effects of exogenous progesterone. She was discharged from her latest reproductive endocrinologist's protocol because she refused to receive any more injections. She said the stress of the fertility procedures was driving her insane.

Her menses began at age 17 (late menarche indicates a weakness of the kidney's reproductive function); they have always been painful. The pain typically lasted from two to 12 days, beginning soon after ovulation and continuing until the first couple days of menstruation. She bled around five days, the bleeding was heavy, dark red to black in colour, with clotting. The menstrual blood got progressively lighter from days one to six, starting off black going to heavy crimson with clots and toward the end became orangey and watery. Then the blood sometimes became brown and scanty at the end, and sometimes remained up to ten days. There was excessive pre-menstrual tension, breast tenderness, and acne. She often suffered from yeast infections and vaginal discharge. She became extremely fatigued around ovulation to the point of physical exhaustion. She had low back pain before and during menstruation. She experienced loose stools and pain with defecation.

Emily had a very stressful occupation. She also stated that she had excessive facial hair, although none was observed. Her fallopian tubes were clear as per her gynaecologist's report. She reported chills, cloudy urine, frequent urination, frequent urinary tract infections, chills, low energy, dizziness, fatigue, excess thirst, insomnia, irritability, unclear mind, anxiety, heart palpitations, fear, sadness, uncontrollable crying, aversion to cold, much phlegm production, nausea, bloating and gas, irregular heart beat, numbness in her arms, cold hands and feet, lack of strength, thin skin, easily bruised, broken blood vessels, dry skin, brittle nails, and low sexual energy. She got dizzy when she stood up and had poor night vision. Her ears rang occasionally. She had extreme emotional liability.

Emily was thin and appeared frail, but agitated. She clenched her teeth and spoke as if she was going to cry. Her husband was always ready to console her. She wasn't sure if she could handle acupuncture because she was "very sensitive to needles." Her pulse was superficial and taut. The kidney aspect of the pulse was very deep and weak.

I diagnosed Emily with liver depression, qi stagnation, depressive heat, spleen qi and kidney yang vacuity, blood stasis, and liver and heart blood vacuity (perhaps due to, but definitely complicated by the stagnated qi and blood). She lived out of town, so we were going to have to devise a treatment plan that would require her presence at the clinic only once per month.

Treatment: *I decided not to try acupuncture on her, but gave her and her husband instruction on dietary therapy, breathing exercises, and massage techniques. I gave her a formula consisting* *of various herbs.*

After the first month Emily reported that she had slightly better energy throughout the entire month (as the qi stagnation was resolving), but she still had frequent night-time urination and a lot of thirst (heat signs). Her pain, though, was diminished. Her pulse was now taut and rapid, but still weak. The second month I gave her a formula consisting of a different selection herbs. This formula spreads the liver qi, strengthens the spleen, nourishes the blood, and clears heat.

She reported after the second month that she had almost no pain before or during menstruation. She continued to experience improvement over the next three months, until no pain was felt on or after ovulation. Her moods improved as the pain diminished.

Emily began charting her basal body temperature after she began her herbal treatments. Her basal body temperature changed from a sawtooth, erratic pattern to a biphasic, healthy hormonal cycle. Six months after her treatment began, Emily and her husband decided to try another insemination. She did not experience the extreme emotional liability with this procedure, and they became pregnant. They are now the parents of a healthy young son.'

Part Three

Further Research

Further Research

This section reveals the broader range of influences on your health, based mainly on scientific research, covering an array of related subjects, which will increase your knowledge of where we are today in our understanding of the disease. Looking at endometriosis in context of modern day society, with its many technical and, so-called medical advances, we are no further in really understanding this disease. But we are gaining an understanding of all the different external influences that are affecting the health of women with endometriosis.

My own research found me being drawn to subjects which at first seemed to go at a tangent, but I soon realised that the information I was finding was indeed very relevant. I began to develop a comprehensive awareness of the opportunism of modern medicine, drug companies, and the economics of health care; as well as the lack of integrity and public health safety surrounding the food industry, personal care products and medicine.

This may seem far removed from your basic needs of wanting to find out how to heal from endometriosis; but I felt this knowledge would empower you to think more deeply about how you actually deal with this disease, as you will be better informed of the subtleties surrounding endometriosis. It would help you realise just how many influences there are on your body that need to be seriously taken into account, if you wish to successfully beat this disease. It would also help you realise that mainstream health care provision does not always have your best interests at heart.

The research for this book took me to some interesting sources of information including:

The World Health Organisation, Greenpeace, US Government Departments, Environmental Health Organisations, medical sources, Endometriosis Advice websites, personal websites with individual insights of the disease, nutrition and alternative health resources, environmental health resources, drug company information, economic statistic information, to name a few.

One of the aims of my research was to get an over-view of this disease, to see if there were any tangible clues, a common thread, as to why women get endometriosis, and why so many women are getting it today. My thinking was that if women, as well as the medical profession, knew (or at least could speculate) what caused it, and then we would know how to reduce the number of women and girls who developed it. To start with I tried looking at the history of the disease and this is what I found.

History of Endometriosis

There is very little information about this disease going back in history. I have found a few snippets of information, but nothing with any meat on it. It may seem irrelevant to find out about this disease historically, but I was personally intrigued to find out how prevalent this disease had been in the past, which may shed light as to why it is becoming so much more common now.

Here are the few facts I did find:

- A recent article from the History Department at the State University of New York notes that endometriosis was described in European history at least 300 years ago
- The first detailed description of wide ranging endometriosis was put forward by Daniel Shroen in 1690
- Austrian pathologist Karl Freiherr von Rokitansky first reviewed endometriosis in scientific literature in 1860. He referred to the disease in his writings as simply "an adenomyoma".
- Prior to 1921, there were only 20 reports of the disease in world-wide medical literature
- In 1927, endometriosis was formally described by Dr John Sampson, when he presented a paper identifying 13 patients in whom the presence of endometrial tissue was observed during abdominal surgery
- The "Encyclopaedia of Medical History" published in 1985 did **not** have a mention for endometriosis

There could be many reasons why there are so few facts about endometriosis in history. Many women may have gone through life with endometriosis, without ever having been diagnosed. This would be especially so with attitudes towards women regarding their reproductive health within the orthodox medical profession, which would have been nearly all male. Historically, if women voiced their concerns over their reproductive health they were usually told that they were being neurotic or else it was all in the head. This situation is still common today.

Many women would have started their families at an earlier age than they do now, in industrialised countries. This would have helped to ward off the onset of the disease, and women were having bigger families in the past.

Until 20 years ago, the only way to do a definitive diagnosis for endometriosis was to undergo major abdominal surgery. This was the case before the advent of the laparoscope and keyhole surgery.

I feel the reason that there are very few facts about endometriosis in history is similar to the reasons we are dealing with today. So few people have heard of it, and I have mentioned some of the reasons earlier. It is therefore poorly publicised, and also poorly funded regarding research.

There probably were many cases of endometriosis in history, but they went undiagnosed. But we are not looking at the same sort of numbers that we are looking at today.

When I was diagnosed with endometriosis the amount of knowledge within the medical profession was limited. The amount of knowledge within the general public was negligible. I had to explain to every friend, relative and acquaintance, what it was I had and what it meant, every time I mentioned endometriosis. I sometimes wished I had a little handbook to give to people to read. It was so tedious as well as soul-destroying, having to describe each time what it was I was dealing with.

A Closer Look at
Possible Causes Of Endometriosis

In the previous chapter we briefly covered the possible causes of endometriosis to act as a reference. The list below is a more detailed look at some of the possible causes.

The retrograde menstruation theory - is the movement of menstrual flow, including sloughed endometrial tissue, back through the fallopian tubes into the peritoneal cavity during menstruation.

Retrograde menstruation has been documented in a variety of surgical studies, and it is estimated to occur in 90% of all menstruating women. So if retrograde menstrual blood is being blamed as the cause of endometriosis, then most women on the planet should have it.

For most women, menstrual tissue debris that enters the peritoneal cavity is destroyed before the tissue can implant in the peritoneal cavity. It is destroyed by the immune system.

If retrograde menstruation is so common, with almost all women experiencing it to some degree with each cycle, why do only 10% to 15% of women develop endometriosis?

The other problem with the theory of retrograde menstruation is that endometriosis has been found in other parts of the body, including the lungs, brain, limbs and even the eyes.

This theory also does not account for the cases of endometriosis found in men who have been taking estrogen as part of treatment for prostate cancer.

Immune system response - In women without endometriosis, ectopic implants of endometrial tissue are destroyed by a variety of immune and inflammatory reactions. These include activation of the cell-mediated immune system, including an increase in the production and activation of cytotoxic T cells that respond to foreign invaders, and the stimulation of natural killer cells.

Inflammatory response - The damage, infertility and pain produced by endometriosis may be due to an over-active response by the immune system to the early presence of endometrial implants. The body, perceiving the implants as hostile, launches an attack. Levels of large white blood cells (called macrophages) are elevated in endometriosis. Macrophages produce very potent factors, which include cytokines (particularly those known as interlukins) and prostaglandins. Such factors are known to produce inflammation and damage in tissues and cells.

Growth factors - Vascular endothelial growth factor (VEGF) is secreted by endometrial cells. Under normal circumstances, VEGF is secreted within the uterus. When oxygen levels drop following menstruation and blood loss, VEGF levels rise and promote the growth of new blood vessels. This process is important for repairing the uterus following menstruation.

When endometrial cells land outside the uterus, however, investigators theorise that this same process occurs with unfortunate results. The cells secrete VEGF when they are deprived of blood and oxygen, which in turn stimulates blood vessel growth. In this case, however, blood vessel growth serves to promote implantation outside the womb.

These are some of the hormonal and biochemical theories, which are linked to immune system imbalances of different types. I do not want to go into more detail on this subject as it is very complex, and I am not medically qualified to go any further, without getting totally lost in the subject. I have focused on the subject of Immune System diseases further on from a laypersons perspective, which is a broader look at the possibility of endometriosis being a breakdown of the immune system as a whole.

Iatrogenic Transplantation Theory - which is the belief that accidental transference of endometrial tissue from one site to another occurs during abdominal surgery. This is highly uncommon today due to advanced surgical management. It does not account for the disease being present in the first place, and does not account for the occurrence of endometriosis in other parts of the body.

Liver Disorder - Some people believe that liver disorders are the key in predisposing a woman to the disease. The liver is a filter of sorts. It detoxifies our body, protecting us from the harmful effects of chemicals, elements in food, environmental toxins, and even natural products of our metabolism. The liver also regulates and removes estrogen from the body through a series of processes. Anything that impairs liver function or ties up the detoxifying function will result in excess estrogen levels. This can happen whether it has a physical basis as in liver disease, or an external cause as with exposure to environmental toxins, drugs, of dietary substances. Estrogen is produced not only internally but also produced in reaction to chemicals and other substances in our food. When it is not broken down adequately, higher levels of estrogen build up.

If for whatever reason, the liver begins failing to remove the estrogen, symptoms such as chronic fatigue and allergies (common in endometriosis) can appear. Another interesting issue is that studies have also shown that the liver is the major target for dioxin and is severely affected by the chemical. A significant number of people exposed to dioxin have been found to have an enlarged liver and impairment of liver function.

Hereditary - Preliminary study results indicate that patients with relatives who have endometriosis may be genetically predisposed to develop it themselves. This theory was suggested as early as 1943. There is research currently underway on this theory. I do feel that this avenue of thought has a stronger case regarding a predisposition for the disease, and not that the disease is passed on from one generation to the next. There will be many, many women who are the only ones in their family to develop this disease. There was no history of endometriosis in my own family.

Thyroid Link - Some researchers believe that some women with endometriosis may be suffering from thyroid dysfunction. In one survey of the thyroid function and endocrine levels (hormones secreted from the glands of the pituitary) of 120 women with endometriosis, it was found that although their routine thyroid tests were normal, the incidence of thyroid autoantibodies was 20% higher than the reported percentage in other women. In some cases the levels of thyroid autoantibodies were consistent with a definite thyroid autoimmune disease. Some of these women were treated with low-dose thyroxin and the women's health improved considerable.

History of Abuse - There appears to be a high incidence of a history of sexual abuse in women who later develop endometriosis. Statistics that have come from a survey by the Endometriosis Research Centre show that approximately 42% of women who responded to the survey with endometriosis suffered from sexual abuse before they developed endometriosis.

Autoimmune Disease
is Endometriosis one of them?

There has been much speculation as to whether endometriosis is an auto-immune disease, so let's look briefly at the different ways the immune system can be impaired or fail.

Different Disease of the Immune System

Autoimmune Disease

The term "auto-immune disease" refers to a varied group of more than 80 serious, chronic illnesses that involve almost every human organ system. It includes diseases of the nervous, gastrointestinal, and endocrine systems as well as skin and other connective tissues, eyes, blood, and blood vessel. In all of these diseases, the underlying problem is similar--the body's immune system becomes misdirected, attacking the very organs it was designed to protect.

Many individual autoimmune diseases are rare, as there are many different types of autoimmune diseases. But as a group, however, they afflict millions of people. Most autoimmune diseases strike women more often than men, particularly affecting women of working age and during their childbearing years.

A Women's' Issue

For reasons which are not understood, about 75 percent of auto-immune diseases occur in women, most frequently during the childbearing years. Hormones are thought to play a role, because some auto-immune illnesses occur more frequently after menopause, others suddenly improve during pregnancy, with flare-ups occurring after delivery, while still others will get worse during pregnancy.

Autoimmune diseases also seem to have a genetic component, but, mysteriously, they can cluster in families as different illnesses. For example, a mother may have lupus; her daughter, diabetes; her grandmother, rheumatoid arthritis. Research is shedding light on genetic as well as hormonal and environmental risk factors that contribute to the causes of these diseases.

Autoimmune Reactions

Autoimmune reactions can be triggered in several ways:

- A substance in the body that is normally strictly contained in a specific area (and thus is hidden from the immune system) is released into the general circulation. For example, the fluid in the eyeball is normally contained within the eyeball's chambers. If a blow to the eye releases this fluid into the bloodstream, the immune system may react against it.
- A normal body substance is altered. For example, viruses, drugs, sunlight, or radiation may change a protein's structure in a way that makes it seem foreign.
- The immune system responds to a foreign substance that is similar in appearance to a natural body substance and inadvertently targets the body substance as well as the foreign substance.
- Something malfunctions in the cells that control antibody production. For example, cancerous B lymphocytes may produce abnormal antibodies that attack red blood cells.

Immune Deficiency Disease

What is an immune deficiency disease?

When part of the immune system is either absent or is not working properly, an immune deficiency disease may result. An immune deficiency disease may be caused either by an inborn defect in the cells of the immune system or an external environmental factor may damage the immune system.

There are two types of Immune Deficiency Disease - <u>Primary</u> and <u>Secondary</u>.

<u>Primary</u> immune deficiency diseases are disorders in which part of the body's immune system is missing or does not function properly. They are caused by intrinsic or genetic defects in the immune system.

<u>Secondary</u> immune deficiency diseases are those in which the immune system is compromised by factors outside the immune system, such as viruses or chemotherapy, toxins and pollution.

* * *

Personal Speculation

Looking at the information above, it is difficult to determine whether endometriosis could be an Autoimmune disease or whether it is possibly a Secondary Immune Deficiency disease. These two malfunctions of the immune system appear to have very similar traits - the immune system is impaired or compromised over time. With Primary Immune Deficiency disease, this is a situation in which the individual is born with the problem and is commonly inherited.

Is endometriosis a condition where the immune system is attacking the self! It seems true that an autoimmune reaction is taking place, when particles of the body are found in areas where they should not be i.e. the endometrium. But in the case of endometriosis, the immune system should be attacking those stray cells, but it is not clearing up the stray cells completely. It is left unchecked, which is why these stray cells go on to develop into endometriosis.

In women who **do not** have endometriosis, but who **do** have stray endometrial cells in the pelvic cavity, these stray cells are cleaned up by the immune system. It has been noted that a very high percentage of women do have retrograde menstruation which will contain endometrial cells, but because their immune system is functioning properly, then this debris is destroyed and not left in the pelvic cavity to go on and develop into endometriosis.

My own feelings are that endometriosis is a Secondary Immune Deficiency disease, which is triggered by outside factors like toxins, dioxins and excess estrogens in the body. I doubt if we will ever find out which one of these is the culprit, and maybe its due to a cocktail of things that are compromising the immune system; but considering so many women with endometriosis suffer from other serious health problems in tandem with their endometriosis, then it seems logical to assume that a compromised immune system is the root cause.

This is a very difficult subject to gets to grips with as the immune system is such a complex system, and when it goes wrong the processes seem just as complicated. I have found a lot of information about autoimmune diseases, but little in the way of hard facts about Immune Deficiency diseases. They are obviously different, but the end results seem very similar to me.

More Possible Causes

We will now cover the more revealing and disturbing research that I have unearthed during my research, concerning environmental health and social welfare. This part covers the subject of the damaging effects of toxins in the environment, and their consequences, as being another possible cause of endometriosis. Leading on from that, we will be covering the topic of estrogen dominance.

I personally did have some awareness about the problems of toxins in our environment before I started researching this book, but I had no idea how vast the problem was. I was not aware how far reaching the affects had spread, or how long it had been going on.

The facts about toxins in the environment are depressing and make very grim reading. All of this information has left me personally very angry, especially as governments around the world seem reluctant to deal seriously at this huge global problem. We do have many other pressing problems globally, affecting many members of the human race, but the urgency to deal with this problem is paramount as it has an effect on every person, and living thing, on this planet.

Just for a bit of light reading I have also included a little insight into the issue of the huge profits being made by pharmaceutical companies in the west? This is especially relevant to those women in the US who have to pay for their own drug treatment for endometriosis, if it is not covered by their insurance.

Living in a Chemical Soup

More than 100,000 chemicals have entered into the market since 1945, and it is estimated that 75,000 of them are still in commercial use. Most of these chemicals remain untested for their safety in humans and other species.

44% of 50 countries surveyed by WEDO (Women's Environmental & Development Organisation) all over the world (1999) report reproductive health disorders as a result of chemical exposure in the work place and other occupational hazards.

The health effects of water pollution are especially severe on women and children. In the Ukraine 13% of the illnesses affecting women and children have been linked to water pollution, and 21% to air pollution.

In Russia pollution has led to doubling of bladder and kidney disorders in pregnant women. In the Ural region, the synergistic impact of a cocktail of chemicals is causing birth defects, tumours, malignant blood diseases and diabetes.

In Uzbekistan, prolonged use of water polluted by pesticides and industry has led to increases in pregnancy complications and birth defects, and a higher incidence of anaemia, and kidney and liver diseases in women.

In the UK government experts found that 12,000 to 24,000 people might die prematurely as a result of exposure to air pollution. The incidence of breast cancer has risen massively, and is now one of the highest in the world. 1 in 12 women risk contracting breast cancer in their lifetime, and there is evidence that this rate increases to 1 in 11 in certain regions of the country.

In the US and other industrialised countries, exposure to dioxin in adults is near levels at which the World Health Organisation warns that subtle adverse neurological and endocrine effects may already be occurring.

Persistent Organic Pollutants (POPs)

POPs are toxic, persistent and bio-accumulative (stored in the body). They are substances of organic (carbon based) chemical compounds and mixtures. These chemicals are products and by-products of human industrial activity that are relatively recent in origin. In the early decades of this century, pollutants with these harmful properties were virtually non-existent in the environment and food. Now this group includes a large number of pesticides, industrial chemicals (PCBs) and unintentional by-products (dioxin, furans).

POPs are persistent and very long lasting in the environment and some of them can be found in the environment after decades and even centuries. They are also subject to global distillation and can migrate from warmer to colder regions.

In half a century of production, the synthetic chemical industry world wide (excluding the USSR) had produced an estimated 3.4 billion pounds of PCBs, and much of it was already loose in the environment.

PCBs were introduced in 1929 and became a huge commercial success, and eventually the chemical engineers synthesised tens of thousands of new chemicals that existed nowhere in nature.

In early assessments, PCBs seemed to have many virtues and no obvious faults. They were non-flammable and extremely stable. Toxicity tests at the time did not identify any hazardous effects.

PCBs quickly found a steady major market and they were used as lubricants, hydraulic fluids, cutting oils and liquid seals. In time, these chemicals also found their way into a host of consumer products and thus into the home. They were used to make wood and plastic non-flammable, they preserved and protected rubber. They became ingredients in paints, varnishes, inks and pesticides.

The term "dioxin" encompasses a family of 219 different toxic chemicals, all with similar characteristics but different potencies. Dioxins are never intentionally produced because they have no commercial value. They are unwanted by-products of thermal processes and of chemical formulations. They will be formed during incineration processes, including municipal waste combustion, vehicle fuel combustion, combustion of wood. Formation also takes place as by-products in industrial processes.

PCBs and Dioxins are transported in the environment in the atmosphere. They can be dispersed in the air either as vapour or in aerosol form, especially during the incineration process.

PCBs were on the market for 36 years before serious questions surfaced publicly about these chemicals. In the meantime, manufacturers kept coming up with new uses.

The first person to recognise that PCBs had become a pervasive contaminant was the Danish born chemist Soren Jensen. In 1964 Jensen, who worked a the Institute for Analytical Chemistry at the University of Stockholm, kept encountering mysterious chemical compounds as he tried to measure DDT levels in human blood. Whatever it was, Jensen found it everywhere - in wildlife specimens collected 3 decades earlier, in the Swedish environment, in the surrounding seas, in hair samples of his wife and infant daughter. It took Jensen more than two years of investigation to identify the synthetic pollutant as PCB.

As other scientists began to look for PCBs, they too, found them everywhere - in soil, air, water, in mud in lakes, rivers, in the ocean, in fish, birds, and other animals. The human population has been exposed to PCBs and dioxins via three pathways - accidental, occupational and environmental.

POPs and Reproductive Health

POPs are highly toxic, and have the potential to injure human health and the environment at very low concentrations, sometimes at the concentration of only one or a few molecules.

Damage caused by POPs to humans and other species is well documented and includes:

- the pathologies of cancers and tumours at multiple sites
- reproductive disorders
- immune system disorders
- lack of development in various body systems such as the reproductive system, endocrine system, immune system and neurological system
- adverse effects to the adrenal glands, the liver and the kidneys
- heart disease
- cerebro-vascular disease
- still births
- behavioural changes such as depression, personality changes
- fatigue
- respiratory diseases

Hormone Disruptors

51 synthetic chemicals have now been identified as hormone disrupters, and at least half, including PCBs, are "persistent" products, in that they resist natural processes of decay. These long-lived chemicals will be a legacy and a continuing hazard to the unborn for years, decades, or in the case of PCBs, several centuries.

Hormone mimics - these same 51 chemicals have been found to disrupt the endocrine system in one way or another. Some mimic estrogen, but others interfere with other parts of the system, such as testosterone and thyroid metabolism.

Man made chemicals scramble all sorts of hormone messages, and they can disrupt this communication system without ever having to bind to a receptor in the human body.

An estrogen mimic may interfere with our hormone regulation in different ways. It may:

- block the pathway so the natural hormone may not reach its receptor site
- it may fit into the receptor site and block the hormone pathway
- it may interfere with the metabolism of hormones or their transport in the body

The affects of POPs and the way they mimic hormones has been discovered to influence or alter many different systems in the body including:

- Multiple reproductive health problems in women
- Miscarriage
- Low sperm count
- Conception difficulties
- Immune System Dysfunction

Dioxins

Just about every member of the general population of the planet, from the moment of conception until death, is now exposed to dioxin-like compounds due to contamination of the food supply.

A spectrum of dioxin-like compounds has been identified in the fat, blood, and mother's milk of the general population. Virtually all-human exposure to these compounds occurs from foods, particularly through consumption of fish, meat, eggs and dairy products.

In the 1950s, dioxin was first discovered as the cause of severe health problems among workers who had been exposed to the by-products of explosions in chemical plants that manufacture certain chlorine-based pesticides. In these accidents, dioxin was formed and released into the workplace environment, causing systemic health problems among workers.

In the 1960s and 1970s, dioxin was identified as a contaminant in the pesticides themselves - the components of Agent Orange - and health problems began to emerge among soldiers and civilians exposed to Agent Orange in the Vietnam War. Subsequent studies showed dioxin was an extraordinary potent carcinogen and caused damage to a variety of organs and systems in laboratory animals.

In the 1980s, the scope of the problem suddenly exploded. Dioxin, it was discovered, is formed not just in the manufacture of a few pesticides, but also in a wide range of industrial processes. The scope of environmental contamination by dioxin turned out to be greater than previously thought. Dioxin was discovered in air, water, and wildlife on a truly global scale. By the end of the 1980s, it was clear that every person in the world is now exposed to dioxin.

Because they are so long-lived and can be transplanted long distances through the atmosphere, dioxins are now distributed on a truly global basis. Inuit natives of Arctic Canada, for instance, have some of the highest body burdens of dioxins, furans, and PCBs recorded, due to a diet dependant on fish and marine mammals from the local food chain contaminated by dioxin from distant industrial sources.

Dioxins in the Body

The effects of dioxin on the body are far-reaching and very damaging. Biochemical studies have shown that dioxins act as powerful "environmental hormones". Like the body's natural hormones, dioxin can cross cell membranes and alter the activity of genes that regulate the body's processes of development and self-maintenance.

Some of the toxic effects on the body of dioxin-like compounds include:

- Modulation of hormones and receptors
- Carcinogenic
- Immune System effects
- Birth defects
- Foetal death
- Male reproductivity toxicity including reduced sperm count
- Female reproductivity toxicity including ovarian dysfunction, endometriosis
- Organ toxicity - liver, spleen, thymus
- Diabetes
- Weight loss

Levels of dioxin-like compounds in the environment have already caused large-scale effects on wildlife populations, particularly fish-eating birds, and marine mammals.

Recent research on laboratory animals shows that dioxin causes effects at lower doses than has been previously thought. This was clearly illustrated by an experiment which found that chronic low dose exposure to a dioxin compound TCDD in rhesus monkeys caused endometriosis.

The Endometriosis Association is sponsoring a long-term study of a colony of rhesus monkeys that were experimentally exposed to varying levels of dioxin. The research conducted by Dr. Rier and colleges shows a clear link between dioxin exposure and development of endometriosis in the monkeys. A shocking 79% of the monkeys exposed to dioxin developed endometriosis, and the monkeys who had the most exposure had the most extensive endometriosis.

While Rier says her work with monkeys suggests one promising theory, she cautions that researchers need to ask what the findings mean. Her own answer? "It means that we have identified and area in need of further research."

The incidence of endometriosis in Belgium is one of the highest in the world; this is considered to be linked to the high levels of dioxin pollution in the area. Dioxin concentrations in breast milk in Belgium are also among the highest in the world.

There are other pollutants in the environment that are having serious effects on wildlife and the health of the public. As well as the estrogen-like compounds that are formed by the breakdown of pesticides, there are also the synthetic estrogens used in birth control pills, and in HRT. These compounds are finding their way into streams and rivers, and are eventually found in the food chain.

The United Nations is currently considering the elimination (or reduction) of 12 of the most damaging chemicals that are Persistent Organic Pollutants. This is to be done through the formulation of an international, legally binding treaty. Nine of these POPs chemicals under consideration are pesticides that have been extensively used in both developed and developing countries. Although many countries have banned these chemicals, they remain stockpiled. In some cases they are produced or used illegally.

Although we do not know the full extent to which the toxins in dioxin, PCBs and synthetic estrogens are having on human health, we do know that their effects are global and represent a great risk to the health of humans, the wildlife and the pollution of our planet.

A Moving Testimonial

I just want to finish this section with an article I found in the Greenpeace magazine 'Voice', which I think sums up exceedingly well the poignant and distressing reality of living with the damage caused by our toxic environment.

A series of meetings have been held in different parts of the world to campaign against chemical toxins. The United States was lobbying hard to try and weaken the first global treaty aimed at banning chemical toxins. At one particular meeting, a calm and soft-spoken American, David Prince, spoke up. He testified humbly but powerfully about the sickness that has blighted the lives of his wife and children. The probable cause is a chemical plant located just a few meters from his Louisiana home. The following is an excerpt from his testimony.

Johannesburg, South Africa

5 December 2000

"When I last attended these meetings, in Geneva, my wife Diane was in remission from ovarian

cancer. Today, her cancer has returned and she is now undergoing a course of chemotherapy.

In recent weeks my daughter who suffers from endometriosis has been told that she will need to undergo a hysterectomy thereby eliminating and chance for childbearing. My oldest son is now doing well after his operation for a deviated septum. However, my youngest daughter and youngest son still suffer from bleeding kidneys and ulcers respectively.

All of the above ailments are primarily due to the fact that out local, state and federal governments are unwilling or unable to stop Condea Vista and PPG from dumping massive amounts of pollutants, as a result of PVC production. These pollutants are in the air we breathe, on a daily basis.

Although there are written laws these industries must follow, our calls for help to state and federal officials are ignored

We know that during negotiations our country has been opposing provisions in the treaty to eliminate the production of dioxin by-products by the chemical industry. Therefore, on behalf of my wife, children, the community of Mossville and myself, I urge you to do what is incumbent upon you; protect citizens of the world from these harmful pollutants instead of protecting the polluters, such as Condea Vista. They claim that they create jobs and build the economy. However, we all know that no economy can be built with dead people

We respectfully ask that you do the right thing, by signing a treaty to eliminate these devastating substances, including dioxin."

* * *

Chemicals in the Workplace

Unfortunately the subject of toxins, chemicals, and pollutants continues to mount, but I feel it is valid information. I have a valuable opportunity here to inform you, the person who is reading this book, who is looking for help, support, advice, information, clues; anything that will increase your knowledge and give you a further insight into the whole subject of the many influences on your reproductive health.

The harmful effects of a few agents found in the workplace have been known for many years. For example, more than 100 years ago, lead was discovered to cause miscarriages, stillbirths and infertility in female pottery workers.

There are now more than 1,000 chemicals in the workplace. These are the ones that have been studied in animals and have proved to have affects on reproductive health, but most have not been studied in humans. In addition, there are 4 million other chemical mixtures in commercial use that remain untested. Physical and biological agents in the workplace that may affect fertility and pregnancy outcomes are practically unstudied. The inadequacy of current knowledge coupled with the ever-growing variety of workplace exposures pose a potentially serious public health problem.

But if you ask the companies involved they will deny that there is any problem, or they say that it is un-proven, or they will say that they are taking all precautions necessary with their work force. These necessary precautions are not being checked however to see how efficient their safety systems are. These companies are satisfied with being 'seen to be doing something', without quantifying if their safety measures actually have any benefits.

There was a recent programme on UK television which highlighted this very issue. The programme was investigating a pharmaceutical company that produced a drug that is given to patients of transplants, to stop them rejecting their transplant organs. These drugs are not toxic to the patients who need them and only take them short-term.

But for the women who worked with these drugs over many, many years, the cumulative effect was to result in serious health problems including cancers and birth defects. The protective clothing was totally inadequate, and women were breathing in the dust given off from the pills during the packaging process. There were many cases of serious ill health within this one factory.

A Closer Look at the Chemical Soup

Xenoestrogens and Estrogen Dominance

It appears that numerous women today are estrogen dominant, and a lot of women over the age of 35 are producing only 50% of the progesterone their mother's produced. This is caused by a combination of factors.

Some of the synthetic chemicals that are finding their way into our food, our water and environment actually mimic estrogen (xenoestrogens), which suggests that these xenoestrogens may stimulate endometriosis. It is excess estrogens in the body, whether natural or synthetic that exacerbates or possibly triggers endometriosis.

The fact that synthetic chemicals can mimic naturally occurring estrogens has been known since the 1930s. In recent years there has been a large increase in the discussion of environmental estrogens in scientific literature as well as in the popular press.

Xeno literally means foreign. So xenoestrogens means foreign estrogens. Some of the 100,000 registered chemicals used in industry and agriculture in the world, have hormonal effects in addition to the toxic and carcinogenic effects I have covered earlier. Some of these xenoestrogens may persist in the body fat for decades.

Could this be why we see so many young girls developing endometriosis? They may have a diet which is saturated in xenoestrogens. They are living in an environment toxic with xenoestrogens. So when they start to produce estrogens in their own bodies with the onset of puberty, the delicate balance of hormones is already out of sync.

The influence on the body of all these xenoestrogens, even for women without endometriosis is a complete disturbance of the delicate hormone system. This leads to what has been called estrogen-dominance.

Estrogen dominance has developed for many reasons, including the widespread use of estrogen-based oral contraceptives, and the widespread use of chemicals in our environment that mimic natural estrogens.

Because xenoestrogens are taken up by estrogen receptor sites in the body, and because the hormones in the body interact with its organs and systems, as well as with each other in highly complex ways, they can disrupt the workings of the body as a whole.

This group of environmental toxins includes hundreds of chemicals including:
- the PCBs used in the manufacture of electronics
- highly poisonous pesticides such as DDT and DDE which is even more toxic

- herbicides
- general plastics used in the home

Some researchers suspect that ethynylestadiol (EE) - the primary estrogen compound in birth control pills - plays a major role. Because EE in the urine of women on the pill is able to pass through water treatment plants, it ends up in our drinking water.

To test the effects of EE and other estrogens on wildlife, researchers raised fish in aquariums which had diluted concentrations either of EE or oestrodiol, the primary estrogen in the animal kingdom. They found that even concentrations of EE as low as 0.1 nanograms per litre of water have a significant effect. Researchers concluded that EE is one of the most potent of biological active molecules.

In May 1993 an article in the British medical journal, The Lancet, researchers in Scotland and Denmark hypothesised that xenoestrogens are responsible for a steady declining sperm count in men. Sperm counts have dropped by more than 50% in some parts of the world since 1940. Meanwhile the rate of testicular and prostate cancer in the US and Europe has tripled in the past 50 years.

A major British study revealed that male fish downstream from sewage treatment plants changed sex as a result of estrogen chemicals which had not been removed from treated effluent.

Some of you may have read about the experiments being undertaken by Dr. Ana Soto. This short excerpt is found at several places on the Internet. I will repeat it hear because it is interesting reading. Dr. Ana Soto, an endocrinologist at Tufts University in the United States, had been experimenting with cancer cells taken from the breast and then cultured. She found they would grow only if fed estrogens. One day, the tests were stopped. The cancer cells continued to grow however, for four months, even when no estrogen was fed to them. Dr Soto then realised that the manufacturer of the laboratory flasks she had been using, had started to use a different plastic - one that, when it becomes warm, releases minute quantities of an estrogen-like compound. Her tissue samples were being contaminated by the xenoestrogens from the plastic flask.

Agriculture uses artificial estrogen compounds to fatten up cattle and chicken quickly. Estrogen stimulates the retention of water giving a heavier weight and tender meat. Some authorities say that artificial estrogen compounds disappear from the urine in a matter of days and the animals are then free of artificial hormones. Other authorities say the artificial estrogens are stored in the fat and then eaten by consumers.

In the 1970s and 1980s there was an epidemic of girls entering puberty at a very early age, as young as 7/8 years old, in Puerto Rico, after eating meat and dairy products with high amounts of estrogens. Some young boys developed breasts.

These are only a few of the thousands of examples that can be found, of the profound effects of pollution caused by toxins in the environment.

Some of the sources of xenoestrogens which are regularly used by the general public are:

- plastics - drinking bottles and plastics used in food packaging
- spermicide
- household detergents
- personal care products
- canned food - found in the plastic coating inside the cans
- commercial raised beef, chicken, pork

- birth control pills
- HRT drugs
- parabens used in nearly all commercial toiletries and cosmetics

As well as these xenoestrogens being a possible cause or trigger of endometriosis, the other health problems that can be caused or made worse by estrogen-dominance are:

- allergies
- breast tenderness
- depression
- fatigue
- hair thinning
- excessive facial hair
- fibrocystic breasts
- headaches
- hypoglycaemia
- increased blood-clotting
- infertility
- memory loss
- miscarriage
- PMS
- thyroid dysfunction
- uterine cancer
- uterine fibroids
- bloating
- fat gain
- gall bladder disease
- auto immune disorders
- risk of stoke and heart disease
- excess estrogen implies a progesterone deficiency. This in turn leads to a decrease in the rate of new bone formation - the prime cause of osteoporosis.

Toxic Toiletries

Most toiletries being used in nearly every home today contain toxic chemicals. These chemicals are used because they are cheap, and in turn it makes for bigger profits. These manufacturers will know about the lethal concoctions they are putting together, but turn a blind eye to it. When these chemicals arrive at the cosmetics factories, they are contained in large containers, and on the containers will be warning labels, including the 'skull and crossbones', denoting that the contents are highly dangerous. And yet these same ingredients go into the finished products, which are then sold to the general public. These products include shampoo, baby bath, lotions, face creams etc.

Over the past decade, scientists have been urgently investigating the effects of low levels of synthetic personal care product chemicals found in our water -- lakes, rivers, and oceans. Scientists around the world have now linked these chemicals from personal care products to a growing global health crisis, causing life-threatening and costly metabolic and neurological disorders.

The US Environmental Protection Agency (EPA) recently reported that they have found synthetic hormone-disrupting chemicals in shampoo, hair colorants, sunscreens, fragrances and pharmaceuticals. These chemicals are washed into our water every day and, as a result, they never go away -- they are persistent because of daily replenishment via bathing, swimming and urination.

Out off the 80,000 plus chemicals used in products today, just a tiny fraction were ever fully tested for toxicity, let alone for their hormone interference potential. Currently, toxicity tests required by the government do not evaluate endocrine disrupting effects, so even so-called "tested chemicals" can have unidentified hazardous health effects.

The US Environmental Protection Agency (EPA) in their report "Pharmaceuticals and Personal Care Products in the Environment: Agents of Subtle Change?" reported that **the chemical preservatives called parabens—methyl, propyl, butyl and ethyl — displayed estrogenic activity in several tests.**

These parabens, which have been approved for use as preservatives in toiletries, are found in thousands of products ranging from sun blocks and cosmetics to baby creams. They prevent the products from spoiling but are also responsible for causing allergic reactions such as skin rashes, swelling and itching. They have been used for decades, and were thought to have low toxicity.

John Sumpter, from the Department of Biology and Biochemistry, at Brunel University in Middlesex, has found that these chemical preservatives are estrogenic, and some of them were able to bind with the estrogen receptor sites in the body. When parabens are administered orally, the parabens were inactive, but applied to the skin, butylparaben produced estrogenic responses on uterine tissues.

These preservatives are even found in natural progesterone creams, including methyl and propyl parabens as a preservative, which rather counteracts the required action of progesterone. This means that these chemicals mimic your body's own hormones and can have endocrine-disrupting action when they are rubbed into your body or washed down the drain into your drinking water. These disruptors interfere with your body's endocrine system: your hypothalamus, your ovaries, and your thyroid—virtually every system in your body.

What is an Endocrine Disruptor?

Endocrine disruptors are chemical substances, primarily man-made synthetics that interfere with the function of the endocrine system. These synthetics may be derived from petroleum or vegetable sources and are created in environmentally unfriendly industrial processes using toxic catalysts and reagents.

These chemicals mimic, block or disrupt the actions of human (and animal) hormones and, unexpectedly, do more damage at low levels of exposure than at high levels. These chemicals can also work in sinister yet subtle ways by disrupting the body's ability to produce adequate quantities of hormones or by interfering with the body's hormonal pathways. One single chemical can affect many parts of the endocrine system. Often minute amounts of several of these environmental hormone chemicals can combine to create effects thousands of times more potent than a single chemical.

The endocrine system regulates every function of the body. It consists of the thyroid, pituitary, and adrenal glands, the pancreas, the ovaries and the testes, all linked to the hypothalamus in the brain. The hypothalamus is like the mainframe computer of the body, sending signals to the glands that provide the instructions for creating hormones, which are the natural chemical messengers that tell your cells what to do.

The various endocrine glands send the messenger chemicals via the bloodstream to different parts of the body where they bind to specific receptors that control all cellular functions. One messenger hormone, estrogen, is secreted by the ovaries and plays a major part in the regulation of menstruation, fertility, pregnancy, and fat cell activity.

When you rub body care products on your body or hair dye on your scalp you can absorb or inhale synthetic chemicals that contain endocrine disruptors which may send false signals to your body's endocrine glands. When your glands are confused they cannot function normally and serious health problems result. In addition, when you bathe, the chemicals your body doesn't absorb are washed down the drain into the drinking water supply, where they can cause a cascade of negative environmental problems.

These endocrine disruptors are affecting algae and other microscopic life, fish, whales and birds. Humans are exposed when they drink the water and eat the fish contaminated by personal care product chemicals. The government has found sunscreen chemicals in fish and human breast milk.

Endocrine disruptors are stored in a body's fatty tissues and do not get flushed out with water, thus they accumulate over the years. It is now recognised that the dramatic increases of breast cancer, non-Hodgkins lymphoma and thyroid cancer have been linked to exposure to environmental estrogens. In the past twenty-five years in the US alone, thyroid cancer has increased more than 45%, with more women being affected than men, and has become the number one cancer in children under age twenty, many of whom suffered from foetal endocrine disruption exposures.

These are some of the Ingredients in most Toiletries

Sodium Lauryl Sulphate (SLS)

Found in shampoos, hair conditioners, toothpaste's, body washes. Strong detergent which can cause eye irritation, permanent damage to the eyes, especially in children, skin rashes, hair loss, flaking skin and mouth ulceration.

When combined with other ingredients, can form nitrosamines, which are carcinogenic. Easily penetrates the skin and can lodge itself in the heart, lungs, liver and brain.

Industrial Use:
Harsh Floor Cleaners
Engine Degreasers
Car Wash Detergents
Laundry Detergents

Personal Care Products:
Toothpaste
Shampoos
Body Gels
Bubble Baths
Facial Cleansers
Baby Wipes
Baby Shampoos & Bubble Baths

SLS can damage the immune system; causing separation of skin layers and inflammation of skin. - Journal of the American College of Toxicology.

SLS is a mutagen. It is capable of changing the information in genetic material found in cells. SLS has been used in studies to induce mutagen in bacteria. -Higuchi, Araya and Higuchi, school of medicine, Tohoku University.

SLS is a potent carcinogen when contaminated with any nitrosamines. - FDA Report .

Fluoride

On one particular tube of toothpaste, there is the following warning in bold faced capitals

"WARNING: KEEP OUT OF THE REACH OF CHILDREN UNDER SIX YEARS OF AGE. IN CASE OF ACCIDENTAL OVERDOSE, SEEK PROFESSIONAL ASSISTANCE OR CONTACT A POISON CONTROL CENTER IMMEDIATELY."

Fluoride is linked to 10,000 cancer deaths yearly. Fluoridation is also responsible for 40 million cases of arthritis, dental deformity in 8 million children and allergic reactions in 2 million people. - Dr. DeanBurke and Dr. John Yiamouyiannis, National Cancer Institute, USA.

Research from St. Louis University, the Nippon (Japan) Dental College and the University of Texas show that fluoride has the ability to induce tumours, cause cancers and stimulate tumour growth rates.

Propylene Glycol (PG) Material Safety Data Sheets warn users to avoid skin contact with this substance, and protective clothing should be worn at all times. It is the cosmetic form of mineral oil found in automatic break fluid, hydraulic fluid and industrial antifreeze, yet is also found in make-up, hair and skin care products, deodorants, and aftershave.

Industrial Use:
Anti-Freeze
Paint
Floor Wax

Personal Care Products:
Shampoos
Hair Conditioners
Hand and Body Lotions
Skin and Beauty Creams
Deodorants

Implicated in contact dermatitis, kidney damage and liver abnormalities; can inhibit cell growth in human tests and can damage membranes causing rashes, dry skin and surface damage. May be harmful by inhalation, ingestion or skin absorption. May cause eye irritation. Exposure can cause gastro-intestinal disturbances, nausea, headache and vomiting, central nervous system depression. - From Material Safety Data Sheets

Talc

This is found in baby powders, face powders, body powders as well as some contraceptives such as condoms. Talc is a known carcinogen and is a major cause of ovarian cancer when used in the genital area. It can be harmful if inhaled as it can lodge in the lungs, causing respiratory disorders.

Isopropyl

This is a poisonous solvent and denaturant (alters the structure of other chemicals) and can be found in hand lotions, body rubs, hair colour rinses, fragrances and aftershave lotions. Isopropyl dries hair and skin, creates cracks and fissures in the skin, which encourages bacterial growth and can cause headaches, flushing, nausea, vomiting and depression.

Imidazolidinyl urea and DMDM hydantoin

These formaldehyde-forming preservatives can cause joint pain, allergies, depression, headaches, chest pain, chronic fatigue, dizziness, insomnia and asthma. Can also weaken the immune system and even cause cancer. Found in skin, body and hair products, antiperspirants and nail polish.

Alcohol

This is a colourless, volatile, flammable liquid that is frequently used in beverages and medicine. When it is used in ingestible products it may cause the body to be more vulnerable to carcinogens.

Mouthwashes that have an alcohol content of 25% or more have been implicated in mouth, tongue and throat cancers.

Most popular mouthwash brands have higher alcohol content than beer or wine and that can be dangerous, even deadly to small children that accidentally swallow mouthwash, according to the Non-prescription Drug Manufacturers Association. Many of the top selling mouthwash brands have between 12.5% and 27% alcohol. Now in alcohol terms that's from 25-54% proof.

Petrolatum & Mineral Oil

This is used industrially as a petroleum based grease component and is also known as liquid vaseline, mineral oil jelly, baby oil and paraffinum liquidum. This substance strips the natural oils from the skin and forms an oily film over the skin, which prohibits the release of toxins. It can also cause photosensitivity, chapping, dryness and premature ageing.

Hair Dye

If you use permanent or semi-permanent hair colours there is a good chance that you are increasing your risk of developing cancer.

Both animal and human studies show that the body rapidly absorbs chemicals in permanent and semi-permanent dyes through the skin during the more than 30 minutes that dyes remain on the scalp. In the late 1970s, several studies found links between the use of hair dyes and breast cancers. A 1976 study reported that 87 of 100 breast cancer patients had been long-term dye users. In 1979, a US study found a significant relationship between frequency and duration of hair dye use and breast cancer. Those at greatest risk were 50 to 79 year olds, suggesting that cancer takes years to develop.

Parabens

The chemicals, which have been approved for use in preservatives known as parabens in toiletries, are found in thousands of products ranging from sun blocks and cosmetics to baby creams. They prevent the products from spoiling but are also responsible for causing many serious health problems along with allergic reactions such as skin rashes, swelling and itching. They have been used for decades, and were thought to have low toxicity. As mentioned above, parabens have estrogenic effects on the body, and parabens are found in nearly all toiletry products. As a result using commercial, chemical based toiletries will increase the levels of estrogen in the body and in turn will add to the further development of endometriosis.

More Estrogen Dominance all Round

Scientists have identified chemicals used in toiletries that mimic the effects of estrogens, that have been linked to estrogens dominance in women, a drop in sperm count in men and an increase in breast and testicular cancers. These chemical toiletries must be avoided, not only to assist with dealing with endometriosis, but for your general health and the health of your family as well.

The women with endometriosis who make the change to natural chemical-free toiletries are reporting that there is a marked improvement in their symptoms. For some women this improvement is noticed quite quickly. The feedback of these improvements includes reduction of general pain, reduction of menstrual pain, reduction of tiredness and a reduction in the levels of general malaise.

Yet another Form of Estrogen

We now need to look at another form of estrogen, and that is the phytoestrogens found in our food. These are specific components in plant-derived foods.

Many different plants produce compounds that may mimic or interact with estrogen hormones. At least 20 compounds have been identified in at least 300 plants from more than 16 different plant families. Referred to as phytoestrogens, these compounds are weaker than natural estrogens and are found in herbs and seasonings (garlic, parsley), grains (soybeans, wheat, rice), vegetables (beans, carrots, potatoes), fruits (dates, pomegranates, cherries, apples) and drink (coffee).

Most of us are exposed to many of these natural compounds through food (fruits, vegetables, meat). The two most studied groups of phytoestrogens are the lignin's (compounds found in whole grains, fibres, flax seeds, and many fruit and vegetables) and the isoflavones (found in soybeans and other legumes). Because scientists have found phytoestrogens in human urine and blood samples, we know that these compounds can be absorbed into our bodies.

Phytoestrogens differ a great deal from synthetic environmental estrogens in that they are easily broken down, are not stored in tissue and spend very little time in the body.

There are differing opinions about phytoestrogens' role in health. When consumed as part of an ordinary diet, phytoestrogens are probably safe and may even be beneficial. In fact, some studies on cancer incidences in different countries suggest that phytoestrogens may help to protect against certain cancers (breast, uterus, and prostate) in humans.

On the other hand, eating very high levels of some phytoestrogens may pose some health risks. Reproductive problems have been documented in laboratory animals, farm animals and wildlife that ate very high (up to 100% of their diet) amounts of phytoestrogen-rich plants.

Even though humans almost never eat an exclusive diet of phytoestrogen-rich foods (even vegetarians), those who consume a diet that does contain a lot of soy are exposing themselves to health risks. There is a great deal of soy products added to every-day convenience foods. Some of these sources are quite surprising including cakes, cereals, biscuits, and sauces. So we are eating a lot more soy than we think we are.

Phytoestrogens behave like hormones, and like hormones, too much or too little can alter hormone-dependent tissue function. For this reason, women with endometriosis need to adjust their diet so as not to include too many phytoestrogen rich foods.

Estrogen Explained

Estrogens are primarily made in the female ovaries and the male testes in humans and other animals. Known as the female hormones, estrogens are found in greater amounts in females than males. These essential molecules influence growth, development and behaviour (puberty), regulate reproductive cycles (menstruation, pregnancy) and affect many other body parts (bones, skin, arteries, the brain).

Estrodiol is the most abundant and potent estrogen hormone. Estrone and estriol are other types of estrogens.

Estrogen is commonly defined as "any of a family of steroid hormones that regulate and sustain female sexual development and reproductive function".

Progesterone

While we are on the subject of hormones we need to look at the other important hormone in a woman' body, and that is progesterone.

Progesterone is secreted by the female reproductive system. Its main function is to regulate the condition of the inner lining of the uterus. Progesterone is produced by the ovaries, placenta, and adrenal glands.

Progesterone levels in the body are very low in the first two weeks of a woman's menstrual cycle. At the point when a follicle is released it rises dramatically until day twenty-one to twenty-three, at which point it begins to fall.

In addition to maintaining the lining of the womb and reducing activity in the other ovary, the progesterone produced each month travels to other parts of a woman's body to fulfil other roles. For example, it protects her from the side effects of estrogen, helping to prevent breast cancer, water and salt retention, high blood pressure and depression. The correct levels of progesterone will also help protect against the problems associated with Estrogen Dominance. Progesterone also induces surges of libido.

When a woman is producing enough of this steroid hormone, she is likely to feel great. It helps her to feel content and emotionally balanced in a number of ways.

When a woman is pregnant the levels of progesterone soar. It is the high levels of progesterone that are produced, especially in the last few months of pregnancy that make many women feel on top of the world and why some women love the whole experience.

The natural hormone progesterone is not to be confused with the synthetic hormones, which are used in birth control pills and hormone replacement therapy. These are called progestogens, progestins or gestins. The effects of natural and synthetic hormones on the body differ enormously. The synthetics do not match the body's chemistry, so the body is not equipped to metabolise them properly.

The use of synthetic progesterone can all too often aggravate some of the problems a doctor is trying to treat, making women moody, irritable and bad-tempered. Natural progesterone, by contrast, tends to make women feel calm and stable.

The actions of hormones are so powerful on the body that you need to make only minute quantities of each, as they are required. For instance, at any moment there may be as little as one molecule of a particular hormone to every fifty thousand million other molecules in your blood stream.

This is why there are such dire consequences when the body is polluted by chemicals in the environment that act as hormones, or when the body is thrown out of natural balance by synthetic hormones used in contraceptives, HRT and drug treatment of endometriosis.

My own body was testament to this. A few years ago I was having irregular cycles and I was having a period roughly every 20 days. I left it for a few months hoping my body would correct itself, but things were not improving. Eventually, I went to my doctor and he suggested I went on the birth control pill for a short time to regulate my periods. I was not happy with the idea, but having a period at such short intervals was not only an annoyance, but I was aware of the need not to have my period too frequent because of my history of endometriosis.

So, I got my prescription, and I took one tablet that evening. The following morning I could hardly lift my head off the pillow. I felt very, very nauseous. I could hardly move. Every time I tried to lift my head I felt really sick. Eventually I had to get up. I dashed to the bathroom and threw up. I could not hold down a small sip of water. I was sick on and off for about 4 hours. I eventually improved, had a cup of tea and threw the bloody tablets away. I decided I would let my body balance itself, and it did in time.

The estrogens and progesterone in a woman's body must be in equilibrium for a woman to remain healthy. In many of us they are becoming more and more out of balance. As a result we are now seeing a widespread rise in many diseases and symptoms for which doctors are prescribing more estrogen.

Hormones are very potent substances. We only understand the very basics of how their complex processes actually work. When the balance is thrown out the body goes into a state of decline, disorder and disease. This is especially true for women, whose bodies have very elaborate hormonal processes. Hormones not only direct and determine her physiology, but also influence her emotional and psychological state. Besides creating a myriad of health problems, hormone imbalance can undermine self-esteem, creativity and a general sense of well being.

Let's recap on the above information just to clarify:

Chemicals

POPs - Persistent Organic Pollutants - this is a generic title for chemicals found in the environment which do not break down by natural processes. The word 'organic' is used because they are carbon based.

There are many of the substances in use, which then enter the environment. The best known are PCBs and Dioxin.

PCBs - Poly Chlorinated Biphenyls - which are found in industrial chemicals and pesticides

Dioxins - toxic chemicals which are unintentional by-products of industrial processes.

The above substances are transported in the environment in the atmosphere, water system and soils.

Effect - Hormone mimics - some of the above substances (chemicals) disrupt the natural hormones of the body

AND

- can actually mimic the hormone estrogen
- They are stored in fat cells in the body so are long lasting.

Hormones

Estrogen - is the naturally occurring female hormone. This is the generic name for a group of estrogens produced in the body

Progesterone - is the other naturally occurring female hormone

Phytoestrogens - these are natural compounds found in plants and are capable of producing estrogenic responses in the body when consumed

Xenoestrogens - are synthetic chemicals and pollutants produced by industrial and agricultural activity. They mimic the action of estrogens, so they disrupt the action of the bodies own hormones. Xenoestrogens can also be called - environmental-estrogens, endocrine-disrupters, endocrine-modulators, ecoestrogens, environmental hormones, hormone-related toxicants, endocrine-active compounds

Toxic Doctors

Countless women are having very bad experiences with their doctors with regard to attitudes. Granted, there are some very good and supportive doctors, nurses and specialists, but it seems that they are fewer in number. I know many members of the medical profession are under a great deal of stress and pressure, but from some of the reports I have read, the attitude of some doctors is simply hostile. This should not be tolerated. You need to report that doctor by filing a complaint in writing and then change to another doctor. Even if doctors are not hostile, many of them can certainly be very patronising. I have found this to be true on many, many occasions. That is why I prefer to look after my own health or see an alternative practitioner.

Being patronised is bad enough. Some doctors will talk to you as if you nothing about your own body. You are the one inside your body, you know what it is doing, how it is behaving, you can intuit some of the problems you are having. And yet doctors tell you that you have no idea about your own health. That is like a dietician telling you that you have no idea what a certain food tastes like, even if you have eaten it!

These are a flavour of some of the feedback messages that have been sent to the website at Endo Resolved regarding women's experiences with their doctor:

> *'The doctor was confusing, rude and a real xxxxxxxxx'*
>
> *'He refused to answer any of my questions and just looked at me with this dirty look'*
>
> *' … he didn't even look at my tests…'*
>
> *'I've had my fair share of doctors that are jerks'*
>
> *'He was belittling, patronising'*
>
> *This is a good one ……………*
>
> *'He then proceeded to tell me that I wasn't trained as a doctor and there was no way that I could understand the treatment or complexity of this disease. That I needed to leave the healing up to him and the other doctors and pharmaceutical companies'*
>
> *…… could not understand the complexity of this disease ………… my god, I think every woman on the planet who has this disease is astutely aware of how complex this disease is …..*
> *THEY ARE THE ONES WHO ARE LIVING THAT COMPLEX EXPERIENCE.*

Now, if you went to see a solicitor, lawyer, architect, banker, or any other professional, they simply would not, could not, and will not, behave in the same manner as some of these doctors. It is totally unprofessional.. So where does the mind-set of some doctors come from. It is probably because they are talking to women and they feel they can get away with it. It is time to fight back and demand respect and compassion. These people are supposed to be working in a 'caring profession'.

May I just point you to the Hippocratic Oath below, which is the oath that every doctor takes upon completion of training. You may want to quote extracts of this oath if you file a formal complaint about your treatment.

Hippocratic Oath — Modern Version

I swear to fulfil, to the best of my ability and judgement, this covenant:

I will respect the hard-won scientific gains of those physicians in whose steps I walk, and gladly share such knowledge as is mine with those who are to follow.

I will apply, for the benefit of the sick, all measures which are required, avoiding those twin traps of over treatment and therapeutic nihilism.

I will remember that there is art to medicine as well as science, and that warmth, sympathy, and understanding may outweigh the surgeon's knife or the chemist's drug

I will not be ashamed to say "I know not," nor will I fail to call in my colleagues when the skills of another are needed for a patient's recovery.

I will respect the privacy of my patients, for their problems are not disclosed to me that the world may know. Most especially must I tread with care in matters of life and death. If it is given me to save a life, all thanks. But it may also be within my power to take a life; this awesome responsibility must be faced with great humbleness and awareness of my own frailty. Above all, I must not play at God.

I will remember that I do not treat a fever chart, a cancerous growth, but a sick human being, whose illness may affect the person's family and economic stability. My responsibility includes these related problems, if I am to care adequately for the sick.

I will prevent disease whenever I can, for prevention is preferable to cure.

I will remember that I remain a member of society, with special obligations to all my fellow human beings, those sound of mind and body as well as the infirm.

If I do not violate this oath, may I enjoy life and art, respected while I live and remembered with affection thereafter. May I always act so as to preserve the finest traditions of my calling and may I long experience the joy of healing those who seek my help.

Written in 1964 by Louis Lasagna, Academic Dean of the School of Medicine at Tufts University, and used in many medical schools today.

Again, do not put up with bad treatment, being patronised or any other form of ill-practise. This will be further detrimental to your health. You need and deserve the best care possible. When there is an external source of support, be it from a doctor, alternative practitioner, or other health care worker, just knowing that you are being <u>supported</u> is a huge benefit to your psyche and healing.

* * *

The Economics and Politics of Reproductive Health

There seems to be a conspiracy of the medical drug companies and medical professionals to maintain the status quo for women's health and information regarding the state of their health. Reproductive health, infertility and HRT is big business and big bucks in the west.

Approximately 600,000 hysterectomies are performed each year in the United States; the estimated overall annual cost of these procedures is over $5 billion. This money is paid by insurance companies or by women themselves if their insurance does not cover it. The most common medical reasons for performing hysterectomies are uterine prolapse, endometriosis and fibroid growths.

Hysterectomy is the second most frequently performed major surgical procedure among reproductive-aged women in the US. In most cases these operations will have been totally unnecessary, a point that has been made by a few enlightened members of the medical profession. But who is going to turn away work like that - its easy money.

According to Dr. Stanley West, noted infertility specialist, chief of reproductive endocrinology at St.Vincent's Hospital, New York, and author of The Hysterectomy Hoax, about 90% of all hysterectomies are unnecessary. Gynaecological consultants to Ralph Nader's Public Health Research Group reached similar conclusions in 1991 in their book, Women's Health Alert. According to Dr. West, the only 100% appropriate reason for performing a hysterectomy is for treating cancer of the reproductive organs.

In 1966 a New York gynaecologist, Dr. Robert Wilson, wrote a best seller called Feminine Forever, claiming the virtues of estrogen replacement to save women form the problems associated with the menopause. He called it 'the tragedy of menopause which often destroys her character as well as her health.' Good God, women have been going through the menopause since the beginning of time - why the hell do we need a member of the opposite sex, who has a financially vested interest, telling us that an event that is totally natural, needs to be confused completely with the use of drugs.

His book sold over 100,000 copies in the first year. A nice little profit there then. And of course this book was published in an era when the general public had total faith in the new shiny medical profession, with all its new drugs, new equipment, and new ideas; and so women thought, or were led to believe that what they read was gospel. Women's magazines of the time promoted Wilson's concept, which gave his ideas even more kudos.

From there, Wilson was able to promote and develop the work of his Foundation, which was set up for the sole purpose of promoting the use of estrogen drugs. The pharmaceutical companies contributed very generous funds to his Foundation, in the region of $1.3 million.

Gynaecologists are among the highest paid members of the medical profession. Women will constantly seek the advice and medical attention of a gynaecologist throughout their lives; ranging from menstrual disorders, birth-control, child-birth, menstruation, reproductive disorders, and infertility. It is a life long journey. In the past, many of these health issues would have been dealt with within the family, by seeking advice from older women, and by using traditional remedies to boost the female system.

Women are now bombarded by propaganda, advertising, scare-stories, contradictions of information and even misinformation. We have cases in the UK were men have set themselves up as medical consultants without any training. Thank God some of them have been caught, but this probably means there will be others.

A vast majority of the public in the west have become lazy about their own health or they do not want to take responsibility. They are loosing the control of their own lives. Doctors have become too powerful in their influence, their decisions, and it has made many of them seem omnipotent. Fortunately, women are becoming wiser and taking control for their own health much more and the health of their families.

Skyrocketing Profits

A recent report by Fortune Magazine indicated that the pharmaceutical industry continues to be the most profitable industry in the US. This will no doubt be the case in other parts of the world too. Overall, the 14 pharmaceutical companies that made it onto the Fortune Magazine report combine to make over $37 billion in profits.

Each of the top pharmaceutical firms had profits exceeding that of the entire Defence/Aerospace industry. The company Pfizer, for instance, almost earned double the entire Defence/Aerospace industry ($4.9billion) by raking in $7.8 billion.

Using the information of the Fortune 500 members as raw data, comparison shows the top seven pharmaceutical companies took more in pure profit than the top seven auto companies, the top seven oil companies, the top seven airline companies, and the top seven media companies.

Health Care in the US

Despite being the most powerful nation on earth as well as the richest, health care in the US is on a par with that of some developing countries.

- People in the US pay on average twice as much for exactly the same medication than does every other nation in the world.
- The US is 24th in overall health care provision according to the latest survey by the World Health Organisation.
- Western European countries, where drugs are often much cheaper, consistently rank in the top 10 for overall health.
- 15% of people in the US lack health care insurance
- Studies have shown that uninsured women with breast cancer are 50% more likely to die than insured women with breast cancer.

The pharmaceutical industry in the US has used scare tactics to try and stop reforms in prescription drug legislation from passing in Congress. One of its claims is that real reform will stifle research and development and make their industry unprofitable. As the figures released by the Fortune 500 show, the industry is making the largest profit margin of any industry in the US, with these profits far outweighing their spending on research and development.

People spend more than enough money to ensure that all Americans have access to high quality health services. Unfortunately, much of what is spent goes to supporting administrative bureaucracies and profits for pharmaceutical and insurance companies. Many insurance companies spend a third of their income on administrative costs and profits.

The profits of the pharmaceutical companies are huge, almost immoral, when you look at the appalling health care provision for people, not only in undeveloped countries, but in the US. These companies are doing all they can to hold onto their profits. They are trying to hold up common-sense legislation which is trying to address an imbalance in health care needs and prescription charges. They are doing all they can to block other countries around the world from developing drugs, especially when it comes to drugs for AIDS treatment.

When you consider the potential numbers of women in the world who have endometriosis, and many of these women may be turning to drug treatment to try and gain some relief from their symptoms, the financial figures and profits for drug companies globally is astronomical.

Conclusion

Before we finish this section I just want to recap on all the different theories, findings, discoveries and plausible explanations as to the possible cause or causes of endometriosis.

Let's add up all the evidence so far. Or should I say clues. We cannot say evidence because none of it is fact as far as we know. A lot of it is conjecture. Like I said at the beginning, nobody really knows what endometriosis is, never mind trying to work out how it is caused. So it is a double whammy for any woman who has it. How can you successfully treat something when you do not really know what the cause is? You need to know the cause of a problem before you can solve it.

Endometriosis is a mystery, but I think this will be a good exercise anyway.

Women with endometriosis are dealing with some, or many of the following:

- immune system compromised for different reasons

PLUS

- hormone imbalances caused by the endometriosis itself

PLUS

- liver function compromised, which can lead to surplus estrogens not being filtered from the body

PLUS

- environmental toxins causing severe changes in the delicate balance of hormones

PLUS

- estrogen dominance caused by many factors in the environment, diet, house-hold and cosmetic products

PLUS

- retrograde menstrual debris not being destroyed by immune system

PLUS

- elevated levels of macrophages (white blood cells) which produce chemicals in the body known to produce inflammation and damage to tissues

PLUS

- VEGF (vascular endothelial growth factor) normally used inside the womb, is secreted outside the womb by endometrial growths, which stimulates blood vessel growth and promoting implantation

PLUS

- Dioxins in the system causing untold damage

PLUS

- additional health problems - cancers, chronic fatigue, ME, Multiple Sclerosis, allergies

- to name a few, which burden the immune system even further. These other illnesses probably develop because the immune system is compromised in the first place - catch 22

PLUS

- Possibility of genetic predisposition to the disease

PLUS

- The other subtle, bodily changes which are too complex to cover here

PLUS

- Stress - stress caused by the pain of the illness, and stress caused by other factors of having this disease, making the disease even worse. Stress caused by the worry and fear of infertility. Adding another layer.

PLUS

- Acute delay in diagnosis - meaning the disease is left unchecked for many years and makes matters worse

To Sum Up.......

Researching this disease from the different angles, dioxin's and xenoestrogens come out as the biggest contenders; as major culprits to the possible cause of endometriosis. They could be the catalyst that causes the breakdown in the immune system which then leads to this particular disease in women with a weakness in the reproductive system. It could be the poison that tips the balance for women whose immune system is already compromised by other stresses on the system.

I do not think we will find a single 'cure' for endometriosis using orthodox medicine, especially as nobody really knows what causes this disease in the first place. It is the same with cancer. Doctors and scientists do not really understand what causes cancer. There have been discoveries as to what external things can trigger cancer like asbestos and radioactive compounds. But what happens in the body to then develop cancer is not understood. Also, why do some people get cancer and others do not, when exposed to the same factors.

When the body goes wrong (becomes diseased) the processes are very complex. In many diseases there is more than a single cause. I feel this is the same with endometriosis. No two women are the same. Their bodies are not the same. Their medical history is not the same. Their environment is not the same. Their diet is not the same. Their genetic make-up is not the same. Their life style is not the same. Their attitudes are not the same.

There are so many women that have this disease now that we have to look at it in context. By that, I mean we need to look at why there are so many more case now in this time in history. Why were there much fewer cases reported in the past. Why is it so common in industrialised countries? Why has it suddenly escalated in the last 15 years or so?

Quite clearly, something has to be done quite urgently about the increasing number of women who have this disease. The sheer numbers of women who have endometriosis around the world is immense.

You have been given an insight into the subjects of pollutants, drug company profits and the economics of health care, for a reason. I want you to be informed as much as possible, without labouring over one particular topic. I wanted to put this disease into a bigger context. I want you to have knowledge, because knowledge is power.

Women need to take more control of their own bodies and their health care. The first step in doing this is to find out more about your own body and what it needs.

All too often, people in the West assume that doctors and the medical profession know what is best for them. The world of medicine does not always have our best interest at heart. Pharmaceutical companies are not always making drugs because they are good medicine; they are making them because they are good money. Modern medicine is run indirectly by drug companies. When business profits enter modern medicine, profits become more important than curative results.

Women need to regain their power with regards to their health and not leave it in the hands of those who do not always care or understand. We used to do this in the past, with herbal medicine and with remedies past from one generation to the next. Of course, we had to deal with the 'witch hunt' in the past, which wiped out most of the knowledge, confidence and power that women used to posses with regard to healing. We now need to reclaim that power and trust that we can care for our bodies, our health and the health of our families, in very gentle and natural ways.

Part Four

Your Journey Towards Health

Your Journey Towards Health

In this last, and most important part of the book, we are now going to take a different journey. We have done the gruelling trek to uncover various facts, insights and revelations surrounding the disease of endometriosis.

We are now going to cover a wealth of significant and meaningful material that is going to support you on your journey towards health. This will be more of a pilgrimage, arriving at a destination where you will have so much more power, confidence and faith that you can defeat this disease and reclaim your life.

What we will be covering

Firstly, I will be going back briefly to the story of my own healing and encapsulate the factors that assisted in my own return to health. These factors were based a great deal on my mind set. I will also cover all the practical things I did with regard to helping my body to heal.

Next, we will look at healing in its broadest sense. We will look at theories, the scientific research, mind medicine, and some anecdotal stories of healing.

Following that, we will look at many different practical things you can do to assist your healing. We will look at the self-help approaches to health and have a quick look at different therapies.

After that follows a list of additional self-help measures you can take to assist you, including some simple changes in your mental attitude.

Finally, there are a few more success stories of healing from endometriosis, where women have used alternative therapies or self help measures.

Then, when we have covered all that I will give you a final clarification, a conclusive summing up of all we have covered. I want to leave you with a deep and trusting sense that you can free yourself from the prison of this disease.

My Own Healing Path

The contents of my own story in the first chapter are more of a mini autobiography, focusing more on the events in my life and how they affected me during the time I had endometriosis. In this section I will now go into more detail of the practical things I did with regard to getting rid of endometriosis.

If you have already read my story, having read this book in natural sequence, then you will know that my journey back to health was not plain sailing. Much of this had to do with circumstances in my life. This will also be true for most of you. You simply cannot stop taking an active part in your life, just to try and focus on your health. Life is not like that as we all know.

I was dealing with some huge basic issues around money, housing and relationships whilst I was ill. My family lived a few hundred miles away and they could not get a grasp of how serious my illness was. I did feel very isolated and alone some times. I did have some very good friends, especially those who stuck by me. But the bottom line is, it is down to you to sort your own life out, especially if you are single. All these things exert huge pressures on you mentally, on your inner resources, and if the pressure is too much it eventually affects your health.

I do wonder how on earth I managed to recover from such a serious, disabling disease, especially as it affects the immune system very fundamentally. But I did, and I put a lot of it down to the fact that I changed my mind set.

Information and Support

To put it more precisely, by educating myself and doing as much informative and positive reading that I could get my hands on, it expanded my mind-set rather than changing it. As well as the reading I did about endometriosis, I wanted to discover more about the nature of diseases and then look at the whole topic of healing.

The more I read, the more I began to realise that there is so much more to find out. That has been the same with the research on this book. The more I found out, I realised that there was even more to uncover.

I did not dwell too long, reading up on the subject of disease. I read enough to give me a basic understanding of the different mechanisms in the body that go wrong to cause ill-health. I read about the many external factors and events in life that can trigger disease.

But my main focus was to find as much as I could about healing, in its broadest sense. I cannot remember all the books I read, but I do remember reading 'Love, Medicine and Miracles', by Bernie Seigel. The anecdotal stories in the book, of people who had recovered from serious illnesses and so called incurable diseases gave me so much hope and inspiration. The driving force and message within this book focused on people's mind-set and their faith that they would recover from whatever serious illness they had.

There were many other books I read that provided support, hope and inspiration. If I can trawl my memory cells I will try and recall some of them. I do still have some of them in my book collection, but many of them I borrowed from the library or from friends.

Some of the ones I remember include:

'You Can Heal Your Life' by Louise Hay
'The Road Less Travelled' by M Scott Peck
'Anatomy of the Spirit - The Seven Stages of Power and Healing' by Caroline Myss
'Mind to Mind' by Betty Shine, who is a healer and clairvoyant
'Mind Waves' by Betty Shine
'Hands of Light: A Guide to Healing through the Human Energy Field' by
  Barbara Ann Brennan

I also purchased many reference books, many of which I still use today. As I had decided on Homeopathy to be the main pivot of my healing I purchased a selection of basic self-books on the subject.

I started using essential oils at this time so I purchased a few books to assist me in the use of essential oils for healing. I also bought books on herbal medicine for women, general books on herbalism, books on Bach Flower Remedies, books on foods for health, books about dietary supplements and so on.

I needed knowledge; I needed support from that knowledge; I needed tools to assist me. I needed as much help as possible. I read magazine articles, even about obscure topics, like reincarnation, near death experiences, healing for animals, the healing power of animals, what is the nature of God, shamanism, paganism, crystal healing, magnetic therapies. You name it, I checked it out. I did not go into depth with most of these subjects, but I wanted an insight into all these fascinating, amazing, revealing and sometimes weird subjects.

Having these books and devouring the information they contained gave me a lifeline. I would highlight some passages that I felt were very poignant. I would go back to some of the information and advice again and again whenever I felt my resolve was slipping. I wrote down some of the key information, or some of the wonderful sayings I had found and kept some of them pinned on the wall for inspiration. It did help, a great deal. Some of these books were like my friends.

Some of the subjects I looked into seemed to 'ring true' to me. I felt an affinity with them. I had already decided to focus on homeopathy to assist me in my return to health, but I also became very interested in the subject of healing and healers.

More External Support

I have already mentioned that I went to see a councillor for a short while, soon after my diagnosis. I went because I needed the emotional support to help me cope with the initial shock, fear and worry. I needed advice and guidance to help me cope.

But going for counselling is not cheap, because it is not a 'one-off' appointment, and to be effective you need to go for a while. I did manage to attend enough sessions with my councillor to help me recover from the initial impact of what I was dealing with.

After this, a friend suggested I tried seeing a healer that she knew about, and that she would like to see this healer as well. So the pair of us went one evening the see this woman healer. She was a lovely woman. Very warm, very down-to-earth, and gave both of us a healing session. I did not know what to expect, what she would say, what she would observe or anything.

My friend had known that I was interested in trying healing as an approach to give me more support. The healer we went to see that evening said she could feel the congestion in my abdomen (I had not told her what was wrong) and that she could feel that my right hip was out of alignment so she did some work to help correct the problem. She gave me a general going-over of my entire body to help clean up my aura, and then left me to rest for a while.

I went to see this healer a few times over the period of about 18 months. I do not know how much she assisted me with the healing process, but simply going to see her was an act of reinforcing my faith that I was in control of my own actions and doing something about regaining my health. I always felt very peaceful and relaxed after seeing her, which I knew was bound to be good for my immune system and me.

About a year later I found another healer who lived closer to home, and I made an appointment to see him. When it was my turn for my healing session, his assistant came and collected me and showed me to his treatment room. Treatment room!!!!! It was more like a ballroom. It was huge. It had plush deep blue carpet and heavy drapes at the huge windows.

He asked me to sit down in the straight-backed chair. I told him the very basics of my health problems and what I was doing to help myself. He proceeded by moving his hands around my body just hovering over the surface. He placed the palm of his hand on my abdomen and left it there for a while. Then he moved up my spine and then started to manipulate my neck. He turned my head from side to side and then stopped. He said that I had a problem area in my neck and that I was not able to turn my head fully round in one direction. I tried to turn my head both ways, and sure enough I could not turn my head fully one-way. It just stuck at a certain point. He then did some very gently manipulation again of my neck and I tried again, and I was now able to turn my head round equally both ways.

He then worked back down my spine and over my abdomen again for about 15 minutes. Then the session was over. On my way out his assistant handed me a book that had been written by this healer. It told the story of how he had obtained his healing gifts. He had been in the Royal Air force in the Second World War, as a fighter pilot. He had had a near death experience whilst in active service and soon after started to notice had had developed healing skills.

His specialism was in back injuries and there were testimonies and thank you letters all over the wall in the waiting room of his house. Some of which I read while I was waiting. This was why he was so focused on my spine and was able to detect the imbalance of movement in my neck. It was a very interesting experience even if the healing was not totally relevant.

I had read that some healers do tend to have a particular specialism or an area that they prefer to work in. For example, there are many healers around today that work only with animals.

I did not see any other healers after this. I could not afford it. They were an added luxury, and I concentrated my funds on my homeopathy sessions and dietary supplements. If I had had the money I would have searched out another healer, because I always felt a great sense of calm and contentment after being in the presence of the 2 healers I did see. This feeling always stayed with me for days afterwards.

To compensate for not being able to afford seeing a healer I would use the relaxation and visualisation exercises I had in my reference books. It was hard to do sometimes, trying to stay focused in the moment, not to let the mind wander, especially when suffering pain.

It is always easier to get into the correct frame of mind, a truly relaxed state, when someone else is giving you a treatment, rather than trying to do it for yourself. You know how luxurious it feels to have a proper massage, or when someone else is giving you a manicure, a facial..... you drift off into a lovely dreamy, relaxed state. That is the sort of feeling you can have when you go for a healing session.

A few years later, after endometriosis was totally out of my life, I had sufficient funds to go and train in Reiki healing myself. This is a form of healing that you can be trained in, that allows you to do self-healing, where you can get into that lovely dreamy relaxed state without effort. I will talk about this in more detail further on.

Internal Support

The internal support I used was mainly by taking a few chosen dietary supplements. The Endometriosis Association recommended these at the time. By becoming a member of the Association I was able to purchase them at reduced price.

The ones I took were:
- Evening Primrose Oil
- Selenium
- Multi vitamin and mineral tablets

That is all I took. I could not afford anything else. Sometimes I had to do without these when money was tight. I did occasionally take Raspberry Leaf Tea.

So it is not as though I spent a fortune on every conceivable supplement, vitamin, herbal concoction and elixir to treat myself. Does this give you any more confidence yet in the possibility of your own healing potential - the fact that I was not spending a fortune on therapies, supplements, expensive organic food etc?

There is a long list I have put together of recommended things you can take to support the system when dealing with endometriosis, which comes later. When deciding what to take, I feel it should be up to the individual. There will be certain supplements that will be more relevant to the symptoms or problems you are dealing with.

Diet

The other form of internal support that helped to regain my health was diet. I had been a demi-vegetarian for years, which means I eat fish and white meat on occasions when I feel my body needs it. I hate convenience food, so most of my diet was based on home made vegetarian food. I did not go to extreme lengths to monitor my diet, to eat only foods suitable for a diet for endometriosis, as there was not the information available. My diet was pretty good by default but not specially focused.

The one thing I had to monitor was which type of food I ate as I had awful Irritable Bowel Syndrome. It took me ages to work out which foods would trigger it. I found that vegetables needed to be either raw or fully cooked. If they were partially cooked as in stir-fry, then the cellulose in the vegetables was not broken down and would upset my insides something awful. If the vegetables were left raw, then my gut could assimilate the cellulose and cellular components. The other key thing that would affect it was coffee, and it still does sometimes.

If I could have afforded it at the time, I would have gone totally organic, but I did the best I could. I used to go to the 'pick-your-own' growers in the summer to get fresh fruit and vegetables. I also grew some of my own produce in the summer growing months.

Today I would recommend to anyone to go organic if they can afford it. The vitamin and nutrients are much higher in organic foods as well as being clear of unwanted chemicals.

Exercise

I strongly believe that having regular exercise helped me a lot, not only with the physical aspect of endometriosis, but also with the psychological side. The fact that many days I forced myself to be active rather than lying up in a little ball of misery helped me to maintain a sense of normality. It stopped me from having the feelings of being 'beaten by this disease'.

Some days were harder than others. Of course some days it was impossible to be active when dealing with my period, but if I could manage it, I would. Well, most days I had to because I had my dog to take out. So most days I would be out walking for at least an hour. At the beginning of my endometriosis when I was very ill my partner took my dog out when I could not manage it. But there were days when I would simply push myself through it.

The other thing I did was horse riding, which I have already mentioned about in my story. It is one of those total escape activities, because you have to concentrate totally. It is so absorbing that I find it impossible to be depressed when riding. I love horses, I love the countryside and I love the buzz. I did all my riding by bartering for it, as it is an expensive pastime.

It is excellent exercise, and the more proficient you become the fitter you become. I found it very beneficial for keeping things moving in the abdomen. There is a natural movement in your pelvis when you are riding caused by the natural gait of the horse. When the horse is doing a basic walk is when you get the most benefit. It causes your pelvis to gently move in a subtle tilting manner, backwards and forwards. I always felt as though everything was getting gently massaged internally, which in turn help to keep things supple, as well as help the blood flow. On average I was riding 2/3 times a week.

These were the main forms of exercise I had, as well as gardening in the summer. I would have been as miserable as hell had I not got out and done some exercise. I think for me it was, and still is, important to get out of the house for my exercise. And yes, I even went riding in deepest winter, when it was freezing cold. My eyes would be streaming after a steady gallop with the harsh raw wind blowing in my face. But I always felt exhilarated afterwards. I felt really alive.

Key Support

Along with my positive thinking, a key support to my healing was my homeopathic treatment. I have described in my story the sequence of events with my use of homeopathy, but I did not include much in the way of detail about this treatment.

I think the first and most important thing to point out here is that I did not view homeopathy as a quick fix measure to getting better. You can use homeopathy for first aid and you can use it remedially to deal with certain symptoms.

It was explained to me by Julia, my homeopath, that to obtain total healing from this disease, in fact any disease, then the process needs to be seen as long term. She clarified that to achieve this, and then layers of healing have to be done. The remedies that are chosen have to work gradually deeper and deeper, to realign the entire system of the body. A quick fix measure cannot do this.

She said that it would take about 2 months of healing for every year I had been ill. In many cases, most of us do not know how long we have been 'ill', when the seeds were first planted. In my case it seems as though things started to go out of sync from early childhood. So if that was the case we had many years of early negative influence, plus the more recent years of ill health to adjust.

I never knew which remedies I was being given. I asked Julia to send my remedies with only the instructions and not to include the name of the remedy. That way I would not go and look it up in my homeopathy book and try to work out why she had given me that particular remedy.

My treatment sessions were about 2 months apart on the average. Mostly I took a different remedy each time, but if Julia felt I was gaining a specific benefit, and fundamental things had changed in my life and my health, then she would use the same remedy again to see if its affects were still relevant.

Homeopathy does very subtle things. Not only does it have affects on your physical being, but also there can be subtle changes that start taking place in your life. This is hard to describe, but it's as though what you are giving off with your psyche starts to reflect back at you. This then has a knock on effect in the circumstances in your life, your relationships, you mental state and your general outlook on life. When these changes take place, your health starts to change. It is all about getting things back into balance. Homeopathy treats the whole person, not just the disease, as with all alternative therapies.

You are the disease. That sounds awful I know. Think about it. It is your body that has gone wrong, and that body belongs to you. That body is you. Your body is diseased and so you are the disease. This awful malfunction has happened in you. It is part of you and you are part of it.

There are millions of other women out there, all of whom have been exposed to very similar external factors like you. They have been exposed to the same pollutants, they will have had their own stresses, and they have got the same biological functions as you. And yet they have not got endometriosis and you have.

This is one of the things I tried to get my head around when I was ill. Why it is NOT ONE of my friends has got this disease. They all live in the same area, live similar life-styles, are a similar age and so on, and yet not one of them has this disease. So why do I. There are subtle, unknown forces, subtle factors that have meant that I would get this disease.

This is why it is hard to conceive that anyone will truly know what causes this disease. As I had said earlier, if we do not know what causes it, how can we fix it? The only way to fix a broken body is to get it to fix itself, and it can. The repair mechanisms of the body are just amazing.

The way the body can seal a cut, all by itself without any instructions from us, is amazing. It can mend a broken bone, again without any instructions. It just does it all by itself using such complex messages, chemistry, and cellular repairing techniques, which we have no idea how they work. We understand the basic processes, but we do not understand how the body does this with no instructions. Its on automatic pilot, guided towards repair and self-renewal. That is the bottom line with homeopathy; it strengthens the body so that it can repair itself.

Why I Think I got Endometriosis
Before we go onto the conclusion about my healing I feel it is important to briefly cover why I think I got endometriosis in the first place. When anyone becomes ill they start to look at possible causes, if there is no obvious reason for it. We all go through a vast range of emotions, trying to come to terms with it; trying to weigh it all up; trying to look at what we had done wrong; trying to see how we had mistreated our bodies; blaming ourselves; feeling guilt; feeling anger.

The initial diagnosis is always a shock, no matter what illness you are told you have. It is the fact that your body has gone wrong. It pulls you up suddenly. You are no longer fit, active, fully functioning in life. Everything starts to change in your life. There is a shift in how you view yourself and your life.

It is not easy to be objective about your own life; to look at your life from a different perspective and be able to analyse why a certain event has happened. Some people are able to, but they are few and far between. Most of us just jump up and down and shout 'Why me!' when something goes wrong.

It can take a long time to work out why a particular event happened; why a certain issue had arisen which was not of your making. In most cases we need the value of hindsight in order to understand it. We are then able to put that event into context. We are able to understand more clearly what the events and circumstances were that led up to a situation.

In my own case, my life had been very busy, in fact too busy. I was under more stress than I realised. I had been working on the arts project for 3 years on a voluntary basis, and having to work part-time in the evenings to bring in some money. In the last year of the project, the other 2 original members of the team had resigned due to circumstances in their own lives. One member had a baby, and the other member moved to the U.S. to get married. So I was left holding the fort. I did enlist 2 new members, but the scope of the project, along with the amount of information to take on board was not easy for these new members to take on.

Consequently it was up to me to co-ordinate, manage and control the entire project. This included grant applications, financial planning, monitoring, and liaison work with different funding bodies and arts bodies, co-ordinating the renovation of premises, buying equipment, publicity, and so on. I was working about 60 hours a week. Some days I would be in the workshop up to my eyeballs in dust and muck, the next day I would be in smart clothing having meetings with people from different official bodies. It was very stressful.

I tried my best to continue with the project for another year, but it was becoming evident that I could not continue with this amount of responsibility and workload mostly by myself. There were problems trying to secure revenue funding, and there was a lot of apathy among people in the community, to get them actively involved. In the end I 'threw in the towel' and decided to wind the whole project up. I wanted my life back.

Around the time I finished the project, the relationship I had been in, suddenly came to an abrupt end for no apparent reason. It was not a deep meaningful relationship, but I was very fond of the guy and we had some good times. He phoned me late one afternoon asking for a favour, to run him somewhere in my car, as he had no car himself. He lived right on the other side of town from me, about 10 miles away. He had more money coming in than I did, and he could easily have got a taxi ………….. I had to decline his request, having weighed up the practicalities; especially as it was, 'can you do this right now', sort of attitude.

He put the phone down, and that was the last I saw of him. He moved to another apartment a few days later, I had no phone number for him. I did not know where he was and could not get hold of him.

I was devastated because I was very fond of him. But he had simply disappeared off the face of the earth somehow. I was more upset than I should have been. It had only been a short term, casual relationship. I could not work out why I was so upset. Then I realised; I was so upset because he had done a vanishing act ………… just like my mother. There was no contact, not even after a cooling off period. Zilch! Strangely enough I have not seen him to this day.

I had many bad dreams after he left. Old memories were being thrown up about being abandoned, like I was as a child. I felt wretched, hollow, betrayed. It was awful. I then started to think about the demise of other relationships. It dawned on me that I had actually finished every other relationship in the past. It was as though I got in there first, before they could finish with me. I never wanted to be abandoned again, was my motive. But when it finally happened the other way round, I was left reeling emotionally.

Therefore the winding up of the project and the demise of my relationship happened around the same time. These were the key events in my life. I can see quite clearly in hindsight how I would have gone down hill emotionally; how my confidence would have suffered by having to give up the project; how my health would have been compromised; how my immune system would have left me vulnerable.

It was about 6 months later that I started to feel very ill and suspected that something deep-rooted had taken place in my system. You know the rest. The speed at which my symptoms developed continues to interest me. The fact that the gynaecologist said I was in a total mess internally after my first Laparoscopy, seem to indicate that the growth and development of cysts and adhesions of endometriosis happened rather quickly. Maybe I was one of those who was symptom free for years until my general health snapped after prolonged stress. Then the symptoms of endometriosis finally forged through my system. I do not know what happened except that after a very rough period in my life, my health went down hill and I knew something serious was going wrong.

The fact that it was a gynaecological disorder that I ended up with is of interest, when looking at my own childhood and my feelings of betrayal by my mother. Again, she has never said she was sorry to this day. I have not actually confronted her, but I have tried to quiz her about that time in her life and she just clamps up.

Consequently, my own feelings and thoughts about parenting and becoming a mother were very distorted. I could only rationalise what the whole experience must be like, based on my own experience when I was my mother's child. The whole concept of being a parent appeared to be a huge burden and would take over your entire life for the worse. That was the message my own mother gave to me.

So in essence, I had a fear of parenting; a fear of repeating history; a fear of being an awful mother; a fear of loosing the freedom of my life. I had spent most of my childhood being passed from 'pillar to post', having one adult after another taking control of my life in different ways. There was the Children's Home, the temporary adoptions, back with my mother for a short while, back to the courts for my Father to gain custody because my mother was going to send me to Boarding School, then back with my Father.

I withdrew into myself as a child. I could not rely on adults to listen to my needs or worries or fears; I felt invisible. These fears and anxieties manifested in later life to give me an illness that focused on my reproductive capabilities. This was my weak spot; the one area of my body that held the tensions and anxieties. When my resolve was at its lowest after all the stress in my life, then BANG, it hit me, HARD.

These were my own personal circumstances. But every person is different. Some victims of endometriosis are very young and you may be asking how can they have enough of life's experiences, to build up into a serious illness. These could be the ones whose immune system is weak by nature; or we could be seeing the evidence of a polluted planet showing up in vulnerable young women whose immune system cannot fight back. We simply do not know.

What I do know, and I think we all know deep down, is that becoming ill is a loud, very loud message from the body to correct the negatives influences on the system. We need to search for clues for the cause of the imbalance. It may take a while to find out what all the causes are, and how to correct them. But when we finally uncover the clues, when we finally listen to our bodies, we are then able to take positive action.

Total Healing

My conviction and driving force when I was ill was towards total healing. I did not want to compromise and simply have relief from my symptoms. I wanted rid of this disease, and to repair this malfunction.

I think it helped me to view endometriosis as a malfunction rather than a disease. A disease sounds like something you caught, something external that has invaded your body. Instead I chose to view it as a malfunction, something that is repairable. The malfunction was a breakdown in a biological system - the immune system. This in turn led to the imbalance of the reproductive system which is reliant on delicate chemical actions and reactions through the hormones.

To Summarise my Healing Process:

- Firstly I saw my illness as an imbalance and I did not focus on it as a disease
- I stayed focused on the long term objective of support provided by homeopathy
- I maintained a positive attitude and mind-set that I could be totally healed
- I looked outside myself for support - through my friends, healers, books
- I did not use any modern drug therapy, which could have upset my system even more
- I continued to get involved in physical activities to help maintain health, both physical and spiritual
- I had an attitude which combined bloody mindedness and optimism
- If my resolve faltered at times and I became upset and depressed, I was not too hard on myself. I allowed myself those times to express my emotions. Holding them back would cause more damage deep down.
- I listened to my intuition - I paid attention to my intuition when it told me not to use modern drug therapy. I listened to the needs of my body on a daily basis. I listened when my intuition told me to have the second laparoscopy, even though I had absolutely no symptoms.

My intuition has served me well on other occasions where it has saved my life or helped me to find missing objects - but these stories are not relevant here.

The action I took to heal myself of endometriosis is not beyond the bounds of the average person. I did not have unlimited financial resources, in fact quite the opposite. I had to compromise on the amount of supplements I could afford. My visits to my homeopath were the minimum necessary to maintain the healing momentum. I had lots of stress caused by life in general.

But I think I am quite a 'tough nut'. I had to stand on my own two feet psychologically, as a young child. I had to be emotionally self-reliant. I think these traits in me helped me to knuckle-down to the task in hand. And yes, I did have times of deep despair. Some of these times were caused by the emotional roller coaster of having such an awful disease. Other times were actually caused by the homeopathy. Some of the remedies can bring up all sorts of deeply buried emotions. But I do think it was very necessary and beneficial to my healing to bring these old wounds to the surface.

I think the bottom line to my healing was my belief that I would get well. I then used tools and support mechanisms to help me do this. If I can instil enough belief in you, then you too will have the confidence and faith to forge ahead and heal yourself of this nightmare.

Lots of Stuff about Healing

Before we go onto the subject of healing I feel it is valid to look at some of the factors within ourselves that leave us open to becoming diseased.

What brings on illness and disease? Every cell in our bodies responds to every thought we think and every word we speak. A lifetime of pervasive, negative thoughts about how we perceive ourselves, others and the world around us weakens the immune system and generates an internal environment in which a disease can grow, thrive and even flourish.

Through illness the body is giving us a message, telling us that something is out of balance. This is not punishment for bad behaviour; rather it is nature's way of creating equilibrium. By listening to the message we have a chance to contribute to our own healing, to participating with our body in bringing us back to a state of wholeness and balance.

The word remission is used to describe a period of recovery, when an illness or disease diminishes. A patient is described as being in remission when their symptoms abate. Yet the word also reads as 're-mission', to re-find or become reconnected with purpose. In other words, disease can diminish when we find a deeper meaning or purpose in our lives.

Remission arises by a combination of responsibility and passivity. It is essential that we take responsibility for our own behaviour, actions, words, thoughts and lifestyle. No one else can do this for us. Taking responsibility means acknowledging that healing comes from within. We can then work with others to find the best way to promote our health.

There is a distinction to be made between curing and healing. To cure is to fix a particular problem and Western medicine is particularly good at doing this, by offering drugs and surgery so that disease, illness or physical problems can be repressed, eliminated or removed. It does play a vital role in alleviating suffering, and is superb at saving lives and applying curative aid. But this only goes as far as being without symptoms in many cases.

This is where we enter the realm of healing. 'If you look no further than getting rid of what is wrong, you may never deal with what has brought your life to a standstill' says a patient in Marc Barasch's 'The Healing Path'. To be healed means to become whole. This is not possible if we are only concerned with the individual part that needs to be cured.

Healing is a journey we all share, for in our own ways we are all wounded, whether the wounds are visible or not - we each have our story. A psychological wound is no different to a physical one, emotional hurts are real and just as painful. Most of us become very good at hiding our wounds, not just from others but also from ourselves. When physical difficulties arise we invariably look for a cure while continuing to repress the inner pain. But when we want to know ourselves better, to find wholeness, then the real journey begins.

This means that we need to look at and question our priorities. Looking at priorities means asking why we are really here, what our lives are about, what gives us ours sense of purpose or direction. Is it just to raise a family, to make money, retire, play with the grandchildren and then its over? This certainly brings joy, but it can leave great emptiness inside, due to unacknowledged longings and dreams.

What happened to the athletic teenager who loved to run across the fields and is now trapped inside an overweight and rarely exercised body? What happened to the paintings you never did, the musical instrument you never learnt, and the novel you never wrote? What happened to the pain you felt when your father died? What happened to the anger you felt towards the uncle who fondled you? Why is it so hard to spend time alone? And why do we spend so much time worrying about things that may or may not happen to us!

Illness confronts us with many of these questions. We have choices: we can take a pill and carry on as before, or we can begin to become whole and become the person we truly wish to be.

- You need to look at your priorities - are you constantly serving the needs of others and not looking after your own needs. Are you spending too much time worrying about the 'small stuff'?
- You need to look at your values - are your values so stringent that they do not allow you to be open minded or flexible in your approach to life. The more open you are, the more that new opportunities will show themselves to you. You will be more receptive
- You need to shift your attitudes - are your attitudes also restricting your growth and your health. Are you holding onto grudges, holding onto old anger, suffering lots of resentment?
- You need to amend your life-style - are you doing things that you know are not good for you - bad diet, lack of exercise, doing a job you hate, trying to do too much?

You need to re-assess and reclaim your life.

It is only when we begin to make changes in our life, that we will be able to accomplish true and valid healing. There is no point building a solid house, if the foundations are not secure.

Your Body is Amazing!

Let us first look at some facts about the body to emphasise the point that the body is indeed amazing.

The brain itself is very, very complex, and most of its capabilities and capacities we do not understand. We only use a small portion of its potential. To duplicate the memory portion would require a computer in excess of the size of the Empire State Building.

If all our muscles pulled together in one direction, we could lift as much as 25 tons. Actually, in times of need, men and women have, without stopping to think about it, lifted weight far beyond what is usually considered possible.

Every day our blood travels 168 million miles. That is 6,720 times around the earth. We have enough carbon for 9,000 lead pencils, and enough calcium to completely whitewash a chicken coop.

Constant Renewal

In just the last 3 weeks, quadrillion atoms, (10 to the power of 15 atoms) have gone through your body and have gone through the body of every other species on this planet. If you do radioactive isotope studies, you can prove beyond doubt that you replace 98% of all the atoms in your body in less that one year.

Every five days our whole intestinal lining is renewed. You make a new liver every 6 weeks. A new skin once a month. Every six months we have a new bloodstream. A complete new set of bones within 2 years. Even our brain cells are replaced. The DNA that holds memories of millions of years of evolution, even that is replaced every six weeks.

These facts left me musing on the whole concept of disease and bodily malfunctions. Why would we replace our old cells with 'newly diseased' cells? Why are we not replacing all our old cells with good new healthy ones? So it seems evident that what is happening is that our cells have memories, and we replace the new ones to be just like the old ones. Not the way that nature intended, but the way WE intended. It is like we are perpetuating our own disease.

We start to enter the subject of our perceptions of reality. That tricky question of - do we make our own reality. I will not go into that topic here. We would need to go into too much depth and we would end up going at a complete tangent.

To continue……..

Can you get a grasp of what I am saying here about us putting back diseased cells in our body, when we have the chance to put healthy new cells into our body? We have conditioned ourselves to respond to memories in a certain way. We become convinced by our diseased state. As long as a person is convinced by their symptoms, they are caught up in a reality where being sick is the dominant input.

We do have infinite choices at every second to alter the shape of our world; our perception of our world. But through old, outdated programming we keep on creating the same old patterns in life. We have conditioned reflexes and responses that are constantly being triggered by circumstances into the same predictable biochemical patterns of disease. Our bodies are a mirror image of our thoughts.

We can heal ourselves beautifully and the body does a brilliant job if it is given the chance. To quote from Deepak Chopra from Quantum Healing,

'……….we already know that the living body is the best pharmacy ever devised. It produces diuretics, painkillers, tranquillisers, sleeping pills, antibiotics, and indeed everything that is manufactured by the drug companies, but it makes them much, much, better. The dosage is always right and given on time; side effects are minimal or non-existent; and the directions for using the drug are included in the drug itself, as part of its built-in intelligence.'

The Immune System

There is an awful lot more to the immune system than most people realise. It now appears that the immune system goes far beyond providing protection for the body from invading organisms simply through chemical processes.

I want to quote a sizeable section from a lecture given by Deepak Chopra, M.D. which is titled 'What is the True Nature of Reality? The Basics of Quantum Healing.

'About 20 years ago it was discovered that our thoughts and our feelings have physical substrate to them. When you think a thought you make a molecule. To think is to practise brain chemistry. And in fact these thoughts are translated into very precise molecules known as neuropathies. 'Neuro' because they were first found in the brain; and 'peptides' because they are protein-like molecules. And thoughts, feelings, emotions and desires translate into the flux of neuropeptides in the brain.

You can think of these neuropeptides like little keys that fit into very precise locks called receptors on the cell walls or other neurons. So the way this part of the brain speaks to another part of the brain is in the precise language of these neuropeptides.

What was found subsequently, which was absolutely fascinating was that there were receptors to neuropeptides not only in brain cells but other parts of the body as well. So when scientists started looking for receptors to neuropeptides in cells of the immune system, for example: T cells, B cells, monocytes, and macrophages - when they started looking at them, they found that on the cell walls of all these there were receptors for the same neuropeptides which are the molecule substrate of thought.

<u>So your immune cells are in fact constantly eavesdropping on your internal dialogue. Nothing that you say to yourself, which you are doing all the time, even in sleep, escapes the attention of the immune cells.</u> Not only that, the immune cells, it was subsequently discovered, make the same peptides that the brain makes when it thinks. Now here we come to a startling finding because if the immune cell is making the same chemicals that the brain is making when it thinks, then the immune cell is a thinking cell. It is a conscious little being.

In fact, the more you look at it, the more you find that it behaves just like a neuron. It makes the same chemical cords that the brain uses for emotion, thought, feeling and desire. An immune cell has emotions. It has desires. It has intellect. It knows how to discriminate and remember. It has to decide when it sees a carcinogen, 'Is this a carcinogen? Should I go after it? Should I leave it alone? Is this a friendly bacteria? Should I go after it or leave it alone?' It has to remember the last time it encountered something. In fact it remembers the last time somebody else encountered the same thing.

Your immune cells can immediately recognise anything that has ever been encountered by any living species. If you are exposed to pneumococus for the first time in your life, your immune cells still remember the last time somebody somewhere in prehistoric time encountered a pneumococus and knows how to make the precise antibody to it. It is not only a thinking cell but it remembers way back into evolutionary history of not only the human species but other species as well. So you ask a good neurologist the difference between an immune cell and a neuron and they will say there isn't any. The immune cell is a circulatory nervous system.

Now if that wasn't enough of a startling discovery, the subsequent discoveries in science have been even more interesting, because when scientists started looking elsewhere in the body they found the same phenomenon. When they looked at stomach cells and intestinal cells they found the same peptides. The stomach cells make the same chemical cords that the brain makes when it thinks. Of course they are not verbally as elite as the brain, in that they don't think in English or Swahili, but nonetheless, they are thinking cells. When you say, 'I have a gut feeling about such and such,' you are not speaking metaphorically anymore. You are speaking quite literally because you're gut makes the same chemicals as the brain makes when it thinks. In fact your gut feelings may be a little bit more accurate because gut cells haven't yet evolved to the stage of self-doubt.

What science is discovering is that we have a thinking body. Every cell in our body thinks. Every cell in our body is actually a mind. Every cell has its own desires and it communicates with every other cell. The new work is not mind and body connection, we have a body-mind simultaneously everywhere.'

I just want to quote one smaller section from this same lecture by Deepak Chopra, to give you another insight, or even a quick reality jolt about the nature of our being, our existence.

'............If you could see the body as a physicist could see it, all you'd see is atoms. And if you could see the atoms as they really are, not through the artefact of sensory experience, you would see these atoms of particles that are moving at lightning speeds around huge empty spaces. These particles aren't material objects at all. They are fluctuations of energy and information in a huge void of energy and information. If I could see your body not through this sensory artefact, I'd see a huge empty void with a few scattered dots and a few random electrical discharges here and there. 99.999999% of your body is empty space! And the .000001% of it that appears as matter is also empty space.'

Deepak Chopra goes on to explain that all this 'empty space is a fullness of non-material intelligence ….. or information that influences its own expression.' The tone of his whole lecture is to knit together ideas about the nature of the mind, the body and the nature of reality. Not an easy range of subjects individually, never mind trying to put them altogether.

Deepak mentions that we have a thinking body and that every cell thinks; this equates to what I said earlier about our bodies being a mirror image of our thoughts. What we think becomes manifest in our lives.

That is all I want to cover on the subject of the immune system. I feel that what Deepak Chopra disclosed is extremely thought provoking with regard to how we perceive and understand the nature of our bodies and how they work. We are still only in our infancy with respect to understanding how the body really works.

What is Healing? – The Science Bit

What we are going to look at now is healing in the traditional sense of the word. Many people will have heard different titles to describe healing. Some of these terms include Spiritual Healing, Faith Healing or Laying on of Hands. I don't want you to go wobbly here and thing 'Oh no, cranky healing stuff'. Do read on. Just wait till you have read the scientific research about healing later in this chapter. I think it will give you food for thought.

I will be talking about healing without it being bound up into any sort of category here. We do love to compartmentalise things as human beings, but I want to keep this simple. The end results, as well as the concepts used in different forms of healing are basically the same to some extent. All healing is done with the best intention, and for the better good of the individual involved.

Healing is not to be confused with Therapies, such as Acupuncture, Homeopathy, and Osteopathy etc. These are all healing in their intent, but not the same as having a session with a healer.

The people who are healers find their skills in many different ways. Some are born with acute sensitivities to the needs of others. They can find themselves doing simple basic healing as children, and will work with the welfare and care of animals.

Some healers suddenly discover their healing abilities after a near-death experience. Others come to healing after serious health concerns of their own. And some people who are sensitive enough can be trained to be healers, which takes many years to achieve. All healers will have done a lot of training to help them do their job to the best of their ability.

Healing in Context

Healing brings about harmony of the body, emotions, mind, and spirit of an individual. Healing is about treating the person who has the disease, and not merely addressing the disease the person has.

Healing is the intentional influence of one person (the healer) upon another living system (the person, animal), without using any known means of intervention.

There are two main methods of utilising healing energy. The first is the laying on of hands over the subject, often combined with visualisations. The other method is through meditation, prayer or other focused intent, again often combined with visualisation. The second method is used to send healing at a distance. Visualisations may include seeing the person in need as whole and well.

There have been many controlled studies of healing, and many of them demonstrate significant effects. These include studies on humans, other animals, plants, bacteria, yeast cultures, cells in laboratory cultures, enzymes and more. Some of these studies were with touch healing, some with hands held near the treated organisms, and some were done from distances of several meters to several miles.

Healers are working with the subtle energy bodies when they are doing healing. Healers report that several interpenetrating, subtle energy fields surround the physical body. These subtle energy fields extend to various distances from the physical body. Though only a few sensitive people are able to perceive these subtle energies as visual halos or auras of colour around the body of living organisms and inanimate objects, many people can sense them with their hands. There are many doctors and nurses who have received some form of training in healing that are able to perceive the auras around people.

Most people who are gifted with healing are not academically or research oriented and have difficulty translating subtle energy perceptions into language that is acceptable to conventional scientists. These problems have contributed to the difficulties of science in accepting reports of healers.

In our modern world we are led to believe that whatever is not perceivable by the outer senses (sight, sound, smell, touch,) or measurable with mechanical, electromagnetic or particle physics instruments, then it must be 'non'sense. But technology continues to move on in leaps and bounds, and more sophisticated equipment that can measure the subtle energies, that are involved in healing have been developed.

Historically, societies around the world have had great faith in healing. In some parts of the world, the healing arts are still seen as valid and are interwoven with the fabric of their society. We in the west have become far too removed from our heritage of knowing how to look after the world and how to look after one another. Scientists are now just beginning to realise that the material, measurable world in which they live and study is not the only form of reality.

Successful Research into Healing

Instances of scientific research in the area of healing are beginning to be taken seriously. There are quite a few experiments that validate the usefulness of healing.

Some of the more interesting results of these experiments demonstrate that the positive results of healing are not down to the placebo effect, while other experiments indicate that the energy is non-physical in nature in that the benefits do not diminish regardless of the distance between sender and receiver of healing.

An experiment using a particular healing technique demonstrated its ability to increase haemoglobin values in the blood. Haemoglobin is the part of red blood cells that carry oxygen. A medical doctor, Otelia Bengssten, MD conducted an experiment with a group of 79 sick patients. Together the patients had a wide range of diagnosed illnesses including pancreatitis, brain tumour, emphysema, multiple endocrine disorders, rheumatoid arthritis, and congestive heart failure.

Laying-on hands treatments were given to 46 patients with 33 as controls. The treated patients showed significant increases in haemoglobin values. The effect was so pronounced that even cancer patients who were being treated with bone-marrow suppressive agents, which predictably induce decreases in haemoglobin values showed an increase. The majority of patients also reported improvement or complete disappearance of symptoms.

Laying-on hands healing has been validated by experiments carried out at St. Vincent's medical Centre in New York. The experiment was carried out by Janet Quinn, assistant director of nursing at the University of South Carolina. The design of this experiment rules out the placebo effect of healing. Thirty heart patients were given a 20 question psychological test to determine their level of anxiety. Then they were treated by a group trained in laying-on hands healing. A control group of patients were also treated by sham healers who imitated the same positions as those who had training. Anxiety levels dropped 17 percent after only five minutes treatment by trained practitioners, but those who were only imitating a treatment created no effect.

Dr. John Zimmerman of the University of Colorado did some work using a SQUID (Superconductive Quantum Interference Device), and has discovered that magnetic fields several hundred times stronger than background noise are created around the hands of trained healers when doing healing work on patients. No such fields are created by 'sham' healers, indicating that something special is happening with the trained healers. The frequencies of the magnetic fields surrounding the hands of the trained healers were of the alpha and theta wave range similar to those seen in the brain of meditators.

Dr. Grad of McGill University in Montreal carried out experiments involving plants and the quality of water being used to feed the plants. Sealed containers of water were given to a psychic healer to hold and others were given to a severely depressed patient to hold. The plants watered by the healer-held water had an increased growth rate and those watered with water held by the severely depressed patient had a decrease in growth rate.

In another experiment involving a psychic healer Olga Worrall, Dr. Robert Miller used and electromechanical transducer to measure the microscopic growth rate of rye grass. The device used has an accuracy of one thousandth of an inch per hour. Dr. Miller set up the experiment in his laboratory and then left, locking the door behind him to eliminate any unnecessary disturbance. Olga, located over 600 miles away, was asked to pray for the test plant at exactly 9pm that evening. When Dr. Miller returned to the laboratory the next day, the test equipment had recorded normal continuous growth for 6.25 thousandths of and inch per hour up to 9 pm. At that time, the record began to deviate upward and had risen to 52.5 thousandths of an inch per hour which was an increase of 840 percent. This increased growth rate remained till morning when it decreased but never to its original level.

More experiments are being done and scientific theories are being developed to describe healing techniques. With increasing interest, along with more sensitive equipment, science will be able to more completely understand and validate the reality of healing.

Human beings, and all other living creatures, have their own electrical-magnetic energy balance. The human body floats in a sea of magnetic fields - those of the earth, moon, sun and other galactic fields. The earth itself has an iron core that generates a halo of electromagnetic energy, reaching far beyond our atmosphere. All life on earth has adapted to and existed in this natural electromagnetic environment for millions of years.

When a trained healer attempts to heal, it has been noted that distinct changes take place in the body's magnetic field. The pulsed bio magnetic signal produced by a healer's hands can penetrate body tissue with ease, a phenomenon which is made use of during magnetic resonance imaging (MRI) diagnostic procedures in hospitals.

The benefits of healing are able to act upon the body at the atomic level. In turn, electromagnetic applications in energy medicine (healing) effect many changes at a cellular level. This results in heightened tissue repair and wound healing, enhanced immune functions and the reduction of inflammation. The actions of healing can also bring about the elimination of allergic sensitivities and the re-establishment of energetic harmony to the body as a whole. In addition, healing often brings a sense of well being and peace - a general uplifting of the spirit.

A Change of Beliefs

To understand how healing works scientifically, we need to have a quantum shift in our thinking, our understanding of physics and our understanding of the universe.

Newtonian physics in the late seventeenth century encouraged us to believe that everything was made up of solid matter and that everything worked on a purely mechanical basis. We have learned over the centuries to base all scientific proof on this Newtonian physical "reality". This approach can greatly weaken our intuitive or psychic powers, because we are always seeking "proof" instead of accepting that sometimes reality spreads beyond the pure mechanics of the universe.

With great scientific discoveries like Einstein's Theory of Relativity in 1905, J.S. Bell's Superluminal Theorem of Universal Connectedness in 1964, and the more recent discovery of morphogenetic fields and connectedness of consciousness by Rupert Sheldrake, our concept of universal energy is continuously expanding.

Quantum physics shows us that we are all energy fields moving and interacting with other energy fields. Kirlian photography has given us scientific proof of these outer energy fields or auras of people, plants and animals. Photographs have been taken by Dr Thelma Moss in the USA of hands sending energy to another for healing. Special cameras have been designed to capture the auric layers of people, showing a specific energy pattern before and after healing. The different frequencies of auric energy have been captured through colours and we can now have an aura photograph showing our true, colourful selves.

While the field of energetic medicine has been evolving since the 1930s, the scientific proof of its validity was not established until the early 1970s in Germany. Today there is ample scientific proof of the existence of the human energetic aura carried out by research at many major universities of the world. We now have instruments which can measure aspects of the human energetic body. Energetic medicine is now taught at medical schools around the world. But energetic medicine is not as well known in the United States, as in Europe, where the field evolved. This new order of reality is now accepted as a property of quantum physics.

It was not until the development of the microcomputer chip in the 1980s that a practical way of correcting the ultra-fine energies of the human system became possible. Prior to that time, the energetic body was only able to be assessed. The complexity of the microcomputer chip made it possible to access and correct ultra-fine human energies in the information field.

It requires a paradigm shift in thinking to move from a see-able, materialistic way of viewing the world, to allowing room for the unseen connection between the physical body and the subtle forces of our spirit and the universe.

A Healing Story

I want to recount this story of healing from endometriosis that I read in Betty Shine's book Mind to Mind. I should rather say that the story found me............ so that I could tell it to you. It is funny how these things happen. I was looking through my old books, looking for anecdotal stories of healing to tell you, to give you more faith in the healing process. I had not looked at some of these books for years. I happened to pick up Betty Shine's book, and the pages fell open <u>immediately</u> to the story I am about to recount for you. I have decided to include the entire chapter and not to summarise it. The italics are the words of the patient.

' .... If I see that medical drugs or hormones are actually causing serious problems without benefiting the patient, I suggest that perhaps the tablets could be reduced or given up for the time being, while healing is being given. Jenny is a case in point; she is also an example of how a positive personality can help to complement the healing process.

A lovely greathearted lady in her thirties with her own printing and design studio in London, Jenny used to suffer badly from frequent migraines, accompanied by bouts of vomiting. The fact that she was unwell when she first came to see me didn't subdue her personality; she's on the large side, and I remember her taking one look at my rather narrow healing-couch and joking about whether she'd fall of!

Jenny had woken one Saturday with ' a thundering migraine, as usual ', but had to go to her office to finish some work for a film premiere that evening. Too ill to drive, she ordered a cab; the driver happened to be Leslie (a friend of Betty's). She warned him she would have to stop several times to be sick. He was very concerned about her and couldn't believe that she was actually going into work; when he delivered her to her office he gave her my business card and said: 'Ring this lady. She will sort you out.'

Even though she was feeling half dead Jenny got straight on to me; she found that even hearing me on the phone made her feel a little better. In fact as soon as Leslie gave her my name and she started thinking about me her mind energy would automatically come into contact with the healing energies around me. We made an appointment for the following week; in the meantime, I told her to sit quiet for a while, and relax and breathe properly. Her migraine didn't go immediately, but she did stop vomiting. She came to see me a week later; I'll let her tell you what happened.

Betty immediately made me feel at ease. She ushered me into her healing-room and asked me to take off my shoes and lie on the couch. She told me to relax and explained that she would place her hands all over my body - starting from the feet - and try to find the cause of these migraines.

Her hands felt very hot and hovered over my tummy. Betty said, 'What are all these scars?' I explained that at the age of sixteen, I had a thirteen-pound growth removed from my womb and that I had had four further operations since then in the same area. IN fact, I had just spent a week in a hospital in Wimbledon as a private patient and had been told that after all these operations my body was not functioning properly. I had endometriosis, and had apparently been suffering from it for a long time. It became worse from time to time and caused a lot of side effects.

I could see that the lining of the womb was in a mess, and very inflamed. When I gave Jenny my diagnosis, she said: 'Thanks! I've just paid a hospital five hundred pounds for that information! And it took them a week to find it out.' Endometriosis is the development of the womb lining, the endometrium, in other parts of the body; no-body knows what causes it, but it can create a lot of pain and misery, and also infertility. Jenny goes on:

I had been taking hormone tablets for about two years and after this last spell in hospital my dosage had been increased. Betty immediately told me that my tummy problems were the root of all my troubles, especially my migraine. I had to laugh, because I had come about my head and in ten minutes Betty had taken me back twenty years to the root of the problem.

At the time I really couldn't work it out, but I kept thinking how the bloody hell did she know about my scars when I was fully clothed? Well Betty told me that she would need six weeks to treat me and I should see her for one hour each Saturday, but she said that she couldn't help unless I stopped taking the tablets.

I knew without any shadow of doubt that, on top of her other problems, the hormone pills were producing an enormous amount of fluid retention. The superfluous fluid was actually pressing on her brain, causing the migraines, as well as making her feel bloated and tire. I didn't think it would damage her health if she stopped taking the pills for a month while we watched her progress; she could always start them again if the healing were not effective. Jenny agreed straight away to stop, but on her way home she started having doubts.

I had been taking these tablets for over two years now and was being treated by a very well known gynaecologist I had a hundred per cent faith in. I decided then and there that I would go back the following Saturday to Betty, but I would continue with my tablets and not let her know. Best of two worlds I thought!

Next Saturday I saw Betty again. Off with the shoes and on the couch. 'Did you throw the tablets away?' Betty asked. 'Oh yes,' I lied through my teeth. Betty put her hands on my tummy. 'Sorry, but I know you haven't. Your body is still reacting to the tablets and I can tell you are still taking them.' I felt such a fool being found out, as well as embarrassed at telling lies. Betty laughed at me as I must have looked so silly. 'OK. I promise to stop from today.'

Betty assured me that she could cure me and that I didn't need the tablets. Even though I believed in her I continued to take them for another week. I thought, 'she'll never know this time.' I think I was frightened to stop taking them - perhaps I subconsciously thought I would start growing a tail.

The following Saturday I was found out yet again. From that day I decided to stop taking the tablets. I put them down the loo. Two weeks passed and already a miracle happened. I hadn't had even one little migraine. That alone was a blessing.

On my third visit to Betty knew that I really had stopped this time. She said I was steadily improving and that she could work better now. I remember that Saturday well. After my hour's healing I felt drained and was so tired. I went home and couldn't stop yawning. I went to bed early that night. I woke next morning fresh as a daisy. I had a nice shower and as I was drying myself - my husband said, 'Christ! Look at that bruise. You look as though you have been kicked by a horse!'

Across my stomach and over my right hip was a huge bruise, as big as a dinner plate. Suddenly I felt a bit scared. I knew that I felt OK, but I phoned Betty and explained what had happened.

As usual Betty laughed and said that the healing was working well. She explained that the bruising was a phenomenon that often appeared. I took this in not really understanding it at all, but knowing that something almost magical had taken place.

Jenny's stomach was apparently all colours of the rainbow! Quite why this bruising occurs I don't know, but it has happened so often that I know that it is always followed by a cure. For Jenny:

That was the turning point. I saw Betty on another three following Saturdays and each week she told me how much better I had become. She didn't need to tell me; I was feeling marvellous. My migraine had vanished and my skin was looking great. I felt so much happier and healthier.

I asked her to come back for a booster every six to eight weeks, to ensure that she stayed well. Soon after this last visit, she had her six-monthly check-up with her gynaecologist. 'I went just for the hell of it,' writes Jenny, 'because I had totally forgotten him. I knew I was well - better than I had been for years.'

I went to his private clinic and he checked me externally and internally. He asked me a lot of questions and told me to get dressed and wait until he called me in. I could tell by his face that he was pleased. He said, 'Well, I am happy to tell you that you are completely clear. I won't stop the tablets, but I will cut the dose down and you can see me again in six months.'

I asked him if it was the tablets that had cleared my problem at long last. 'Well yes - but it is very unusual for this complaint to disappear altogether. You must be a lucky lady.'

I told him I had taken hardly any tablets since I last came out of hospital. I told him exactly what had happened since I saw Betty. I was shocked to learn that this was nothing new to him He made no real comment except to say that the most important thing was that I was well and that I was clear of the problem which had plagued me for twenty years. He never finished writing the prescription.

Five years have passed now and still no sign of the migraine. I have had no tummy pains and I feel extremely well and happy.

One or two interesting points come to my mind about this story. Firstly the fact that Jenny's healing could not be done until she stopped taking the hormone treatment, which was seriously affecting her health. The bodies' natural healing processes could not be activated by Betty until she did stop the hormones.

I was angered by the doctor's use of the word 'complaint' to describe what should be medically called a disease. That was exceedingly patronising.

Jenny's healing was complete, it was a total cure. The endometriosis never came back, and in Jenny's words, 'she felt better than she had done in years.

My own experiences of training for self healing

It was a couple of years after I was totally free of endometriosis, that I finally decided to pursue my own path to discover more about healing and to receive training in the healing arts. Mind you, before I found this particular healing tradition, I did not know that a person could be trained in healing. I always thought that healers were born to this skill or else they suddenly discovered the skill after a life changing experience.

The thought of being trained in healing was alien to me. Leading up to my own training, I had been reading a few magazine articles here and there, talking about different healing techniques, how to use them and how you could train up to do this, that and the other. I was also noticing many adverts in the back of those glossy health magazines and spiritual magazines, about training courses, and attunements, to become a healer.

I was very cynical. These adverts described things like 'Get your healing training at the mystical ruins of Macu Pichu', or 'Find your hidden energies for healing in the ancient land of Egypt.' It all sounded very flaky to me; just a load of hype; a good opportunity to milk people who are easily influenced by this marketing. So, initially I ignored it.

But it would not go away. I kept coming across circumstances, where this whole healing and training thing kept cropping up in my life. I was finding more written evidence to back it up; I was meeting people in one-off situations who had done the training; then the final push came when a friend rang me up, and said she had seen some advertising for training in Reiki Healing at a local alternative training centre. The fees were very reasonable, the venue was close by, the times of the sessions were convenient, and so I thought I would go for it. It would not cost me much to find out about this training in healing stuff.

I had the phone number of the woman who was running the course, and it was advised for prospective participants to ring first and discuss it; to get a feel of what it was about, and whether it was the right thing to be doing. So I rang up, and after my discussion on the phone, I could not wait to get started. Suzanne, the woman who was to give us our training, sounded so down to earth. There was nothing 'fluffy' about her; none of the airy-fairy, head in the clouds nonsense. She explained it so simply and with such relish that I just had to do the training. So in the end the training found me. The old saying goes, 'When the student is ready, the teacher will appear'.

So what is Reiki?

Reiki has been around for thousands of years under different names. Some believe that it was in every day use in lost civilisations. Reiki is really two Japanese words - Rei and Ki. When translated, the word Rei has many levels of meaning, one of which is universal or transcendental. Ki means vital or life force. This 'life-force' energy has many other names within different cultures throughout the world e.g. 'Chi' in Chinese, Prana' in Sanskrit and 'Bioplasmic energy' by Russian scientists.

All living things on earth have a 'vital force', an unseen energy to the naked eye. There is photographic evidence in the form of Kirlian photography which has produced 'before and after' pictures of a Reiki healers hands and shows significant changes in the amounts of energy being emitted. Those people gifted with the ability to see subtle energies have also reported that Reiki energy appears to be completely different to other forms of hands-on healing energy, being more powerful and of much higher frequency. Psychics who work with Reiki Masters have also confirmed that the energy appears to have its own intelligence and goes where it is most needed without being guided.

Kirlian photography can also show the energy fields around ordinary people, plants, and animals. The halo of colour that shows up around the silhouette of an individual, or plant, will be of different colours, depending on the condition of health or the state of mind.

Therefore we all have this vital energy, but we do not all possess the extra energy that comes from being attuned to Reiki. Being attuned is a process, an initiation and a 'rite of passage' into the healing energies of Reiki. You can read about Reiki, you can have Reiki treatments, but you will not have the Reiki energy unless you have the attunement. One Reiki Master has used the analogy that it is like the person is a small portable radio that can only pick up local stations. Once that person has been attuned to Reiki, the circuits are upgraded and the person is now able to pick up international wavelengths. It is like having a switch turned on that tunes you into much more subtle energies that are floating around the entire cosmos.

Scientists know about this invisible energy. Some people have tried to invent equipment that will harness its power, and some have succeeded. But you will not hear about this because governments have quashed the findings of these brave inventors. Lives have been threatened. Inventions have been destroyed. To tap into this free and inexhaustible supply of energy would throw global economics into complete disarray.

And the most outrageous thing is that the technology that these governments are suppressing would provide unlimited sources of non-polluting energy for all. I will not go any further with this topic for fear of going off on another tack. Suffice to say, it is another conspiracy we have to deal with someday, and soon, before the planet chokes to death. If you wish to find out more read 'The Coming Energy Revolution' by Jeane Manning.

This universal energy is the same energy we can use in healing, but there is something added to it. That 'something' is unknown, but it is very spiritual and special. But like I said, we need someone who has already been honed into this energy to then pass it on to the next person.

The main points about Reiki are as follows:

- Reiki is very simple to learn and requires no special knowledge or experience
- There is no need to enter into an altered state before giving treatments
- Reiki goes to where it is needed most and always treats the root cause
- It is complementary to all other therapies and conventional medicine
- It is totally safe - you can never 'overdose'
- It reduces healing time dramatically
- It does not require a diagnosis

To be attuned to Reiki, it is done in three stages. The first stage allows you to treat yourself. The second stage allows you to treat others and to send healing at a distance. It also allows you to send healing energies to events in your life. The third level is when you become a Reiki Master, and this is the level where you are able to then pass on the Reiki energy to others and to attune them to start practising Reiki themselves.

I have been attuned to all three levels, but the final level of Reiki Master was not done with full training, as my attunement was given to me as a gift from a woman I met while I was travelling in the Far East. It was a wonderful gift, but I do not feel that I have received sufficient training and understanding to start training others.

I will not go into any more detail here. If you want to find more about Reiki it is on the Internet, and there are many books on the subject. I do endorse the idea for any woman who has endometriosis, to get herself attuned to the first level so that she can give herself self-healing treatments.

To Sum up on the Process of Healing

We have covered a lot of ground here on the subject of healing, even going on a slight tangent with regards to universal energy.

Up to this point I have said quite a bit about self-responsibility for your own health. That does not mean you have to struggle all by yourself; we are all here to help and co-operate with one another. Seeking and accepting help of a healer or health therapist is part of helping oneself. Quite often, seeking outside help is a huge relief and helps to aid the start of the healing process. You are taking action, and that action is empowering.

"Thanks so very much for the two healings I've had from you. After the first one I really slept much better, and I think I'm finally cured of my endometriosis which caused me big problems. The flow has stopped after bleeding severely for eight years. I can't thank you enough. I won't be needing surgery."
L. P., Stockholm, Sweden.

* * *

Support, Support and more Support

We have now finished with the research and background material to this book. I have told you my own story, and included my own observations why I think I developed endometriosis. I have also given you an insight into a few topics that do not seem directly relevant, but I feel it was valuable information for you to have; ranging from the detailed facts regarding pollutants to the fascinating nature of healing. I have tried to give you as much knowledge and information to re-enforce my message that you can conquer endometriosis. All that follows now are the practical things you can do to aid and assist you on your own journey back to health.

The first thing you need is support. That support can be in many forms. It can be through healing, natural therapies, vitamins and supplements, controlled diet, meditation, counselling, reading positive information, talking to friends, joining support groups and many others. Let us start then to look at all the different positive things you can do.

Natural Medicine and Therapies

Many natural therapies, which have been an integral part of health care in other societies for centuries, are relatively new to the developed world. Pharmaceutical drugs and medical technology have dominated modern medicine in the West, but there is a growing interest in therapies that treat the patient as a whole.

Today's interest in complementary and alternative medicine appears to be worldwide. Popularity in the West has grown steadily since the 1970s, accelerating in the 1980s and 1990s. A survey in 1993 showed that one in three American adults used some form of non-conventional therapy. The survey also revealed that more visits were made to complementary practitioners than to conventional doctors.

Traditional Chinese medicine, Ayurveda, and chiropractic therapies attract an enthusiastic following in the US, but therapies widely used in Europe, such as homeopathy and aromatherapy, have been slower to gain ground. Following public demand and anticipated cost benefits, several American health insurers now cover some complementary treatments. In Australia complementary and alternative medicine is even more popular that it is in the US. Nearly half the population is said to use at least one remedy not prescribed by a doctor; over one-fifth have visited a complementary practitioner.

In Europe, studies suggest that between one-third and one-half of the adult population has used some form of complementary medicine at some time. In the UK, a nation-wide survey in 1991 suggested that 20 - 30% of the 30,000 general practitioners in the National Health Service would like complementary therapies to be more accessible within the state system.

Disenchantment with Modern Medical Science

Improvements in living standards, and medical and scientific progress, have raised people's expectations of health and health care. The discovery of drugs such as penicillin and mass-inoculation programs has diminished the terror of once-fatal infectious diseases. Medical technology in the form of X-rays, brain scans, and keyhole surgery, and scientific miracles such as heart transplants and the saving of premature babies seemed to give doctors godlike power over life and death.

But the blind faith many people placed in medicine was shaken when so-called wonder drugs revealed unpleasant or dangerous side effects. Bacteria and viruses developed resistance to many of the drugs that once annihilated them, and pharmaceutical drugs and invasive surgical procedures failed to deliver the complete cures that were, perhaps unrealistically, expected of them.

It is undeniable that particular areas of modern medicine have provided great improvements in health care for certain illnesses. But despite this progress, cures for cancer and AIDS remain elusive, and long-term diseases such as endometriosis are difficult to diagnose yet alone to treat.

Many people now turn to complementary and alternative therapies because they believe them to be more effective for their condition than conventional medicine. This is beginning to be the case for women who have endometriosis. The emphasis on treating the whole person and allowing patients to play an active part in maintaining health is also attractive. With its focus on partnership, holism, and self-healing, alternative and complementary therapies can therefore seem like a more accepted approach.

What is Alternative Medicine?

Alternative medicine is any form of practise that is outside of conventional modern medicine. It covers a broad range of healing philosophies, approaches and therapies.

Complementary Medicine

When alternative medicine or therapy is used alone or instead of conventional medicine, it is called 'alternative' medicine. If the treatment or therapy is done along with or in addition to conventional medicine, it is referred to as 'Complementary Medicine', as the two practises complement each other.

Holistic Medicine

Many of the alternative practises deal with the mental, emotional, and spiritual aspects of health, in addition to the physical body. The name 'Holistic Medicine' comes from the connection between mind and body. Holistic practitioners treat the whole person as opposed to the individual organs where symptoms occur.

Alternative medicine is made up of a rich variety of techniques and medical systems that for the most part, are still unfamiliar to the majority of the public. They are therefore, an 'alternative' to what most people are using when they need health care.

Much of what is labelled alternative medicine comes from other cultures or from ancient healing traditions. The use of herbs as medicine is an ancient practise found all over the world. Acupuncture comes specifically from ancient China and has been documented as being in use as early as 2697 B.C.

The World Health Organisation estimates that between 65 and 80 percent of the world's population rely on traditional medicine as their primary form of health care.

What is the Difference between Alternative and Conventional Medicine?

Generally speaking, most high quality alternative medicine is founded on six core principles and practises that differ from the principles and historical practises of conventional medicine. They are:

- The healing power of nature first, with technique and technology second
- Patient centred rather than physician centred
- Do no harm - many alternative medical systems are rooted in the principle of 'always use the least drastic harmful therapies first'. This means that alternative medical providers, in general, choose techniques and therapies which are the least invasive or harmful to get the desired result
- Results generally take longer - but this ensures long term health and not a quick fix it
- Use of natural and whole substances
- Higher standard of health

The whole area of alternative medicine is becoming more mainstream in western society as a means for people to take care of their health, for reasons including:

- the realisation that, contrary to previously held beliefs, conventional medicine (the medicine of antibiotics, surgery, chemotherapy etc.) cannot solve all of societies health problems
- the growing acceptance that health is more than just 'the absence of disease' and involves more that just the physical body
- the growing body of scientific research, as well as public awareness, that many alternative medical treatments are more effective, more economical, and less invasive and less harmful than conventional medical treatments

An Overview of Different Therapies

I have chosen therapies which I felt were most relevant for the treatment of endometriosis. There are many different therapies available, which are of use for many conditions and health problems, but I have focused on treatments which I feel will be most effective for the treatment of endometriosis.

Herbalism

Herbal medicine is the treatment of disease using medicinal plants, both internally and externally, to restore the patient back to health. It is a system of medicine that relies on the therapeutic qualities of plants to help the patient by enhancing the body's own recuperative powers. It is a natural method of healing based on the traditional usage of herbs coupled with modern scientific developments.

Though there are those in the orthodox medical world who ignore herbal medicine, even condemn it, the constituents of herbs have provided the blueprint for many of the most effective and widely known drugs used today. 'Orthodox' medicine has its roots in herbal medicine.

Orthodox medicine is based on drugs isolated from plants, or more often manufactured in the laboratory. The herbalist advocates the use of the whole plant as a gentler and safer way to restoring a patient to health.

There are two different types of substances found in medicinal plants, and both have an important role to play in the healing process. The primary healing agents are the active ingredients which early chemists were interested in extracting. The other compounds in the plant determine how effective the healing agent will be by making the body more of less receptive to its powers. Most healing plants contain several active substances, one of which will be dominant, and it is this one which influences the choice of plant by the herbal practitioner when making up a prescription for the patient.

The secondary healing agents are just as important, because without them the active substances could have a totally different effect. It is the natural combination of both types of substance in the whole plant that puts the patient back on the road to health.

All medicinal plants contain a range of different therapeutic agents and therefore have a variety of different actions, related to the combine effects of these components.

The main actions of herbs

- they relax tissues or organs which are over tense, predominantly muscles and the nervous system
- they stimulate 'atonic' tissues or organs (those lacking tone) such as sluggish bowel or liver
- they cause constriction of over relaxed tissues, such as muscles, blood vessels and mucous membranes producing excessive catarrhal secretions
- they promote elimination of wastes and poisons from the liver, bowel, kidneys and skin. This particular action is of real benefit for endometriosis sufferers, to help eliminate toxins and unwanted estrogens
- they help overcome infection by stimulating the body's defences and also have direct antiseptic, antibiotic and anti-fungal actions
- they enhance the circulation of blood and lymph
- they aid appetite and digestion and stimulate the absorption and assimilation of nutrients from our diet
- they soothe mucous membrane and thereby reduce irritation and inflammation - another good benefit for endometriosis relief
- they regulate the secretion and action of hormones and where necessary promote hormone production - this action will benefit endometriosis relief by balancing the hormone levels

Herbal remedies are less harmful than chemical drugs. However, it is a mistake to suppose that natural means completely safe in any amount. There are some herbs which must be treated with great respect and care. Some of these herbs can be toxic if taken incorrectly.

Consulting a Practitioner

You need to find yourself a qualified Medical Herbalist. Qualified herbalists should have been trained in all the basic medical sciences - physiology, anatomy, pathology and different diagnosis, and should also have passed a theoretic as well as clinical exam in physical examination techniques and diagnosis. They will also have studied plant pharmacology.

The first session will take about an hour and subsequent visits about 15 to 30 minutes. Details of any conventional medication you are taking will also be recorded to ensure compatibility with the herbal remedies prescribed. The practitioner will carry out some simple tests or give you a physical examination. Based on the practitioners' conclusions, you will be prescribed one or more herbal remedies. Treatment may also include advice on diet and exercise.

The active properties within many plants have been used by many women with endometriosis to provide great relief from symptoms, to help the body detox, and to counteract the synthetic estrogens taken up by the body from pollutants and household chemicals. Herbal remedies are powerful. There are some gentle herbal remedies you can try for yourself, which you can buy over the counter, to help with the symptoms of endometriosis. To use herbs for real healing you are advised to see a qualified Herbalist.

Success with Herbalism

'I am extremely happy that I am able to share my life story with those who are looking into alternative treatment for endometriosis. For seven long years I went from specialist to specialist, treatment after treatment, only to be told there was no hope for me. I was diagnosed with Endometriosis. I did not know what to do. My marriage was falling apart. Than one day my co-worker told me about the herbalists at South Hill Herbs, who were treating with herbs. At first I thought, herbs and fertility, what do they have in common? I was desperate so I went to see the herbalists. After having had consultations and being given the herbs that were prescribed to me, I went home not convinced that would happen, but I tried. I had the notion that only medical professionals can help such a problem. To my surprise three months after my visit I was pregnant. My family life changed drastically. My husband and I are happy raising our little boy. My message to those with suffering from is to never give up hope.'

-Margaret, Amsterdam, Holland

* * *

'After 13 years of having to take anti-inflammatory medications for my menstrual cycle, I was not able to function without them. After a ruptured ovary, surgery and extreme endometriosis, my options for a "normal" life involved taking the pill along with an experimental drug that would tell the body it was in menopause or pregnancy, or I could have a hysterectomy.

I used an herbal formula from my herbalist regularly for six weeks. I was two weeks late with my menstrual cycle, so I figured that the formulas were not working either. To my surprise, when I did have my period, I didn't have to use any anti-inflammatory medication. I experienced only one day of cramps that were about 1/10th of the severity that they normally were. Furthermore, I didn't become as sick with nausea or diarrhoea as I usually do. I have been suffering with this problem for many years while thinking that it was never going to go away unless I had a hysterectomy. Certainly, at only age 26, that procedure held its own complications and repercussions!

I am very grateful for the opportunity to try an alternative approach that really works! Thank you for my life back!'
Monica

Aromatherapy

Aromatherapy is a form of healing that utilises the natural aromatic aspect of plants - the essential oils - both for their scent and for their inherent medicinal properties. These aromatic oils can be found in a wide range of species and are extracted from the seeds, bark, leaves, flowers, wood, roots or resin according to the type of plant.

The term 'aromatherapie' was first coined in the 1920s by the French perfumier Rene Gattefosse, who became involved in extensive research into the medicinal properties of aromatic oils after discovering by accident, that lavender oil was able to speed up the healing process of severe burns and prevent scarring.

Although the word 'aromatherapy is new, the knowledge and use of aromatic and essential oils for healing purposes reaches far back to the very heart of the earliest civilisations. The ancient Egyptians employed aromatherapy oils four thousand years ago. The Greek and Roman culture was renowned for its emphasis on the benefits of aromatic bathing and adornment, while the Chinese and Indian traditions still use aromatics extensively as part of their herbal medical system, as well as for ritual purposes. It was only during the last century in the West that the use of home remedies underwent a decline as a result of the scientific revolution and the development of the modern drug industry.

The word 'aromatherapy' can be misleading, because it suggests a type of healing which operates simply through our sense of smell. The fragrance of essential oils is an important part of their overall nature, but only one aspect of it.

In an aromatherapy treatment, essential oils interact with the body in a variety of ways. When massage oil is prepared with essential oils and rubbed on the skin, the essential oils are quickly absorbed through the cell tissue and into the bloodstream to be transported throughout the body. They can then interact with the organs and systems of the body directly.

Massage is the main method used by professional aromatherapists because it ensures a good absorption of the essential oils and is a very relaxing and healing experience in itself. Different essential oils have different properties so a mixture of oils may be used in an aromatherapy treatment.

Scientists working in a number of different fields around the world - doctors, professors of medicine, chemists and biologists - have carried out laboratory tests which prove that essential oils have the ability to prevent the proliferation of harmful bacteria. Most essential oils have antibiotic, antiseptic, anti-viral and anti-inflammatory properties to a greater or lesser extent.

The naturally derived antibiotics, found in essential oils act slowly, and only kill the unwanted bacteria or viruses; they also stimulate the body's immune system to strengthen resistance to further attack.

Properties of different oils

Stimulating oils

(for low blood pressure and lack of energy)

Basil, black pepper, cardamom, ginger, peppermint, pine needle, rosemary, thyme

Relaxing oils

(for emotional or physical tension)

Cedarwood, bergamot, camomile, clary-sage, cypress, frankincense, jasmine, lavender, neroli, rose, sandalwood, ylang ylang

Anti-inflammatory/Healing oils

(especially beneficial for endometriosis sufferers)

Benzoin, bergamot, camomile, frankincense, geranium, lavender, myrrh, patchouli, rose

Anti-spasmodic oils

(for period pains, muscle cramps, also beneficial for endometriosis sufferers)

Black pepper, cardamom, camomile, clary sage, fennel, ginger, jasmine, lavender, marjoram, nutmeg, orange, rosemary

Anti-depressant oils

Basil, benzoin, bergamot, geranium, jasmine, lavender, neroli, petitgrain, rose, ylang ylang

You will note that many oils have more than one benefit.

Although aromatherapy will not be able to provide a cure for endometriosis, (not as far as I know) it can act as a support to the entire system. It is well known that many oils will help to boost the immune system, and will help to keep infections at bay.

Some of the properties of essential oils are very beneficial for endometriosis sufferers, including the oils that have anti-inflammatory and anti-spasmodic properties. There are many other uses for essential oils for endometriosis sufferers including:

- deal with insomnia and aid sleep
- relaxing oils to help with stress
- using anti-depressant oils
- detoxifying - to assist the release of toxins from the system
- relieve pre-menstrual tension

The use of aromatherapy would act as a good support for any woman suffering with endometriosis. You can use the oils in bath water, and have a soak last thing at night using an oil to aid with sleep. A hot relaxing bath with oils is of great benefit when dealing with severe menstrual cramps.

I would suggest that you purchase a few basic essential oils to have around the home. Lavender is the key oil to have as it has so many uses and benefits. Always purchase good quality oils, and try to get ones which are organically grown if you can. You only need to use a few drops of oil at a time, so they will last quite a long time. Keep them stored in a cool, dark place. There are plenty of small hand-books and more comprehensive books available to give you guidelines on which oil to use and for which purpose.

Over the years I have found aromatherapy to be very beneficial for both health and beauty purposes. For those women who do not want to use commercially produced body and face creams because of the negative chemicals they contain, you can make up your own preparations using essential oils. I personally use Almond oil as a base oil, and then add whatever essential oils I choose, to make up a body oil and a bed-time face oil.

You can use essential oils in the following ways:

- mixed with a carrier oil for massage
- added to bath water
- added to a carrier oil for a healing/beneficial body oil
- burned in a vaporiser so that the essential oils are vaporised in the atmosphere - good for colds and flu
- steam inhalation - good for chest infections
- compress - for cuts, wounds, bruises, swellings

Homeopathy

Homeopathy is a therapeutic method of medicine in which very dilute doses of natural substances (plant, animal, mineral) are administered to a patient to treat symptoms that would be induced in a healthy individual by ingestion of that same substance.

Homeopathy stimulates the body's own defences to correct illness and allow symptoms to dissipate. The minute doses of drug substances used in homeopathy do not cause any side effects. Homeopathy can be used for short term (acute) illnesses and long term (chronic) illnesses.

The healing method of homeopathy looks at each patient and develops a remedy or treatment plan strictly for him or her. It invokes the powers of healing inherent in individuals (our Immune system) to develop a successful therapy. The more one knows about the patient, the symptoms, likes and dislikes, what makes them better or worse, it helps in developing a 'symptom picture' of the patient that can lead to a successful treatment.

The principles of homeopathy have a lot in common with our present understanding of immunisation. To prevent us from catching smallpox, a vaccine is prepared which is a mild form of the virus that causes the disease. The principle is that introduction of this small amount of the virus in our body system will set out our body's defences so that when the actual virus shows up, our body will have enough barriers of fighting power to prevent the virus from entering our body.

Part of the theory of homeopathy, the body is said to be integrated by a 'vital force', which maintains it in a state of health. If this force is put under strain, illness can result. Symptoms of illness are seen by homeopaths as signs that the body is using its natural powers of self-healing to fight back. Homeopathic treatment seeks to stimulate this self-healing process rather than to suppress symptoms.

Acute symptoms such as pain, heavy bleeding, mood swings, bloating, pre-menstrual symptoms and bowel upsets can be treated effectively with what is called an acute remedy. These can replace the need for painkillers, laxatives, sedatives and anti-depressants. Some examples of commonly used acute remedies are Magnesium Phosphate, Camomile, Helonias, Sepia and Cimicifuga.

There are over 400 different remedies for abdominal pain, each one being quite specific to include: location of pain, length of pain, type of pain, time of day of worse pain, and so on. This is why it is not advisable to self treat, and you need treatment from a qualified Homeopath for accurate remedies to be prescribed.

Consulting a Practitioner

Practitioners may be homeopaths who are not medically qualified or conventional doctors who practise homeopathy. The practitioner will ask you about your medical history, diet, lifestyle, moods, likes and dislikes, as well as the nature of the medical problem you are seeking help for. A classical homeopath (see below) will also identify your 'constitutional type'. The 'constitutional type' is identified through a persons individual physical, intellectual and emotional traits. Asking many questions about your habits, fears, food preferences, personality attributes, the way different weather and seasons affect you, does this. By doing this, homeopaths can prescribe some remedies for the ailment and some to support the person's constitutional type.

The practitioner will try to match your symptom picture with those catalogued in the homeopathic 'repertories', which include 2,000 to 3,000 remedies, often stored on a computer database. The skill lies in prescribing the remedy that fits your individual type and condition. Advice about diet and lifestyle may also be given.

You will be asked to report and reactions and changes in symptoms at your next visit, and your prescription may be altered or adjusted necessary. With self-limiting conditions, practitioners say that improvement should occur after the first few doses of the correct remedy. Long-term conditions that have developed gradually, require longer treatment, and can take a few years. Once signs of improvement show, the remedy dose may be tapered off and eventually discontinues. A variety of remedies may be used in complex cases.

There are no side effects with homeopathy, but symptoms may briefly worsen after treatment. Homeopaths claim that since the body is healed from the inside out, deep-seated conditions may be temporarily replaced by more superficial ones. For example, as asthma improves, eczema may flare up in its place.

Classic Homeopathy

Classic homeopaths prefer to find a single remedy that matches the patient's constitutional type and symptom picture, and will treat with single doses of that one remedy. This approach depends on identifying the similimum - the match - which may not happen on the first visit. The practitioner can identify if it is the correct remedy by the feedback from the patient on any changes that have taken place. It may take two or three remedies before the right one is found. This is the approach that was used in my own healing using homeopathy. The remedies acted very deeply within my system, which assisted to bring up old emotional wounds that were hindering my healing process.

Homeopathy is a vast and complex subject. It takes 4 years to qualify as a homeopath, which includes working on 'live' cases during training. There is a lot of discussion between the patient and the homeopath, to reveal the true nature of that person and their illness. So there is need to trust the homeopath and feel comfortable with them.

There have been many successes of the use of Homeopathy with endometriosis as well as treating infertility and general menstrual problems. Many women have gained great relief from their symptoms of endometriosis, and some women, like myself, have totally defeated the disease.

Success with Homeopathy

'Jane started her career in conventional medicine, managing one of the busiest hospital operating theatres in London. When she fell ill, conventional medicine failed her. In desperation she went to a homeopath, who cured her of a serious gynaecological condition - endometriosis. She was so impressed that she trained as a homeopath while she was still running the operating theatres of the Wellington Hospital, eventually leaving to become a full time practitioner herself, working in Brighton, London and Milton Keynes. Jane said, "Homeopathy is a complementary medicine. It works on its own, and also with other medical treatments, be they conventional, or alternatives like Alexander therapy, reflexology or cranial osteopathy. "I treat people holistically, encouraging them to appreciate the importance of tackling health with nutritional improvements as well as using homeopathy. Increasingly I have to treat patients who come to me quite ill after extreme regimes of antibiotics or steroids or other toxic drugs. I believe that homeopathy is probably one of the most evolved and effective methods of healing, because it doesn't just treat, it cures. It is very understandable that its growing popularity and success are causing the pharmaceutical

companies some concern.'

* * *

'My family and I have all been greatly helped by Krista Voysest and homeopathy. In 1995 I was diagnosed with endometriosis, I failed to respond to hormone therapy and because I had had two c-sections, my insurance informed me that they would not cover surgery because the risk of a medical emergency was too great. I did not have the money to pay cash for surgery, so I began to resign myself to a life of spending most of my time in so much pain I could not function. At this point, a friend introduced me to Krista. She found the right remedy for me, and I began to improve immediately. My endometriosis has been entirely cured, and I am in better health than ever.' **--T. Liu / Anaheim, CA**

* * *

'Mrs T. came with endometriosis and excruciating back, stomach and period pains, and was due to have a hysterectomy. The first treatment brought some relief from the pains, but she also experienced stomach bloating and carpal tunnel in her left wrist (she had had this ten years before - return of old symptoms). Over the next 9 months there were many changes - the bloating and the pain disappeared, but headaches and depression returned. The headaches then disappeared, but she had terrible sciatica for a while. Then period pains stopped. One year later they returned with a vengeance, but after one treatment they disappeared and she was finally free from pain. One very exciting result - the consultant changed her mind about the hysterectomy - she said an operation was no longer necessary!'

* * *

'There is a huge amount of anecdotal evidence that says it (homeopathy) does work. Louise Hamilton, a 29-year-old human resources officer from Clapham in London, had endometriosis. She endured 15 years of crippling pain and has had three operations and hormone treatment to alleviate her suffering without success. Eventually, the pain got so bad she could not walk. "All I could do was lie on my left side - I could only work for three hours a day." For the past 18 months she has had homeopathic treatment and is now free of pain. "I'm convinced it works. I suffered for 15 years and now I feel so good I've not had to see my homeopath since last May'

Acupuncture

Acupuncture is part of Traditional Chinese Medicine and has been practised in China for thousands of years, but became widely known in the West only in the 1970s, when its use as an anaesthetic received sensational press coverage. Practitioners insert fine, sterile needles into specific points on the body as a treatment for disorders ranging from asthma to alcohol addictions, but most often in the West as a means of pain relief. Now one of the most well-known and most widely accepted Eastern therapies, acupuncture is increasingly practised in a simplified form by medical doctors.

Acupuncture is an element within the Traditional Chinese Medicine health system, which includes herbs, acupressure, exercise, and diet. Fundamental to Traditional Chinese Medicine are the concepts of yin and yang, opposite but complementary forces whose perfect balance within the body is essential for well-being. Yin and yang are components of qi (also known as chi), which is the invisible 'life energy' that flows through meridians (channels) around the body. There are 12 regular meridians running up and down the body in 6 pairs. They are mostly named after the main internal organs through which they pass.

The even circulation of qi around the body is essential for health. Disruption on a meridian can create illness at any point along it. There are about 365 acupoints along the meridians at which qi is concentrated and can enter and leave the body. It is possible to affect the circulation of qi at these points, and acupuncturists insert fine needles to stimulate or suppress the flow.

Consulting an Acupuncturist

On your first visit, the practitioner will take notes on your lifestyle and medical history, and assess your condition using the 'Four Examinations' of Traditional Chinese Medicine - asking, observing, listening and touching, in which the most important test is taking the pulse. This is a skilled method of checking the rhythm and strength of all 12 meridian pulses. To aid diagnosis, the practitioner may examine other parts of the body. They will then discuss treatment options, which as well as acupuncture, often include advice on diet and lifestyle, and may involve herbs.

The treatment involves lying on a treatment couch, after removing any clothing covering the needle sites. The site depends on the disorder and whether the flow of qi is to be 'warmed', reduced or increased. Several acupoints may be used: those on the hands and feet are often treated, but sites on the back, abdomen, shoulders, and face are also widely used.

The practitioner inserts the needles to a depth between an ⅛th to 1 inch depending on the position of the acupoint being treated. A treatment often involves a combination of acupoints; usually 6 - 12 needles are used, varying according to the type of acupuncture and condition being treated. Acupuncture needles may be left in position for a few minutes, as little as a few seconds,, or as long as an hour. At the end of the session they are withdrawn swiftly and gently, usually painlessly, without bleeding, and leave no trace on the skin.

Treatment times vary greatly, from 30 to 90 minutes, depending on how long the needles are left in position. The initial consultation will probably be the longest. Most conditions require between 10 to 20 sessions, depending on the patients age and how long they have been suffering from the condition.

A growing number of doctors now practise 'medical acupuncture', usually for pain relief. For pain relief, Acupuncture may release painkilling endorphins. It may also trigger nerve 'gate control', in which pressure messages reach the brain faster than the messages of pain, but more research is needed in this area. Generally speaking, there seems to be a lot of success with acupuncture to relieve pain.

This particularly benefit will be of interest to those who suffer a great amount of pain with their endometriosis. It would be advised to seek out an acupuncturist to discuss treatment for this particular problem. I personally know of one acupuncturist who has successfully treated various patients with endometriosis, and has great success not only in reducing the pain, but has also eliminated the disease for a number of women. This was seen as a long term plan of treatment, and like all alternative treatments, involved raising the levels of 'life energy', and in turn supporting the immune system to fight the disease.

Success with Acupuncture

'After 7 1/2 years of trying with all fertility options including in-vitro I gave up and a friend recommended Acupuncture for my horrible symptoms. I went to acupuncture for 2 months three times a week and she changed my cycle to where I did NOT have any symptom ie, heavy bleeding cramping etc. and told me to try and conceive. We got pregnant the first month. Just another option which worked great for me. Best of luck. T '

Successful pregnancy with Acupuncture

'Rosy, aged 38, used the Billings method of natural contraception for four years before actively trying to conceive. After eight months and no success she visited a gynaecologist who diagnosed grade 2 endometriosis. She had always suffered from very heavy and painful periods with a lot of clotting but had taken this for granted as 'normal' for her. After reading an article by a fellow endometriosis sufferer, she cut out wheat, dairy and caffeine from her diet. Although this was not easy, she was very determined and noticed an immediate improvement – her next period was lighter and less painful. On the recommendation of a friend she started going to Zita for acupuncture and after weekly treatments through one cycle she conceived her daughter Agnes, who is now 16 months old'

Chinese Herbalism

Chinese Herbalism is another part of the Traditional Chinese Medicine system. The Nei Jing (Yellow Emperor's Classic of International Medicine), dating to c. 200B.C. - A.D. 100, is the earliest known document to set out the principles that underlie Traditional Chinese Medicine to this day. It emphasises the ideals of moderation, balance, and harmony, which are central to the ancient Chinese philosophy of Taoism.

Western medicine, introduced to China by 16th century missionaries, gradually threatened to overtake traditional healing. However, the establishment of The People's Republic in 1949 led to a revival of herbalism, acupuncture and other ancient medicinal skills, known collectively as Traditional Chinese Medicine. In China, Traditional Chinese Medicine is now taught at universities and practised in all hospitals alongside Western methods. Its popularity is growing fast in countries with large Chinese communities, such as the US, the UK, and Australia.

The key principles of Chinese Herbalism are the same as for Acupuncture, based on the need for balance between yin and yang. When the dynamic of yin and yang in the body is disturbed and either one becomes excessive, disease or emotional problems follow. Factors that may provoke a disturbance include infection, accidents, emotional state, poor diet, pollution, and even the time of year and weather conditions.

Herbal remedies are used to rebalance these forces within the body. Herbs are classified under five elements according to taste, each of which denotes a medicinal action: sweet, sour, bitter, pungent, and salty. The opposing yin/yang qualities of hot and cold are also linked with the action of specific herbs. Each herb is said to work in specific organs and related meridians.

The Chinese herbal practitioner has a choice of nearly 6,000 herbs, a few mineral and animal components, and hundreds of different formulas. Herbs are usually used dried rather than fresh, with prescriptions often taking the form of a loose tea. The herbs are rarely prescribed singly, but are generally taken as a formula - a standard prescription may have 10 to 15 herbs with a history of treating a particular pattern of disharmony. Each herb in the formula has a different role. Practitioners often adapt a basic formula, adding other herbs to suit the patient's age, constitution, and pattern of disharmony.

Consulting a Practitioner

The initial consultation may take as long as an hour. Your health is assessed by means of different diagnostic techniques. These include observation of all the visible evidence of your state of health, particularly the tongue, the tone of your skin and hair, and the way you move. The pulse is checked for quality, rhythm and strength. The practitioner asks about family history, habits, body functions and any symptoms of poor health.

The diagnosis hinges on your unique pattern of disharmony. The initial consultation last about an hour and subsequent sessions about 30 minutes. Some conditions, especially chronic, long term complains may require several months of treatment, with consultations every 4 - 6 weeks.

Success with Chinese Medicine and Acupuncture

In a letter (1993) to the Endometriosis Association, one patient wrote: "Several years ago I was fortunate enough to be pointed toward Edie Vickers, the acupuncturist associated with the Institute for Traditional Medicine in Portland, Oregon. At the time, I was adamant that under no circumstances would I subject myself to Danazol. Through regular acupuncture and Chinese herbal treatments, I was able to delay my second endometriosis surgery for a year and a half, at which time the technology and knowledgeable and experienced doctor were available to take care of the majority of my problem via surgical technique. At this time I was 37 years old...I am now 41 years old and consider myself lucky that I still have my uterus, have never taken Danazol or Lupron, and my pain is reduced to ibuprofen-relieved cramps lasting no longer than 18 hours a month...I think the herbs are greatly helpful and I always felt they were really working well. Chinese medicine takes patience, faith, and time, and sometimes lifestyle changes--but, in the final analysis, it works."

Naturopathy

Also known as 'Natural Medicine', naturopathy developed in the late 19th century, founded on an ancient belief in the power of the body to heal itself. Naturopathy believes that the body's natural state is one of equilibrium, which can be disturbed by an unhealthy lifestyle. They look for underlying causes of a problem rather that treating symptoms alone, combining diet and non-invasive therapies where possible to stimulate the healing process. Naturopathy is practised throughout the Western world and some of its principles have been adopted by conventional medicine.

Some aspects of naturopathy have common ground with other ancient holistic health systems. The term 'naturopathy' was coined in 1895 by Dr. John Scheel of New York, but the system grew out of the 'nature cures' popular in 19th century spa towns in Austria and Germany. These emphasised the benefits of hydrotherapy, fresh air, sunlight and exercise.

Modern naturopaths believe the body will always strive toward good health, or homeostasis, and that the body is its own best healer. They maintain that many factors, such as unhealthy diet, lack of sleep, exercise, or fresh air, any emotional or physical stress, pollution in the environment, even negative attitudes, allow waste products and toxins to build up in the body and upset self-regulation. This in turn can overload the immune system and weaken the vital force, the body's innate ability to maintain good health.

Naturopaths believe that symptoms such as fever or inflammation are signs of the body's self-healing powers at work, and advise against suppressing such symptoms, since that can cause the disorder to 'go underground', becoming chronic and causing further degeneration. Rather than treating symptoms directly, naturopaths work to improve underlying health so that the patient is less susceptible to infection.

Naturopathic treatments are as non-invasive as possible. Some practitioners specialise in a particular approach, which other draw on a wide range of techniques. Some of the most commonly used treatments include clinical nutrition and fasting (diet is very important part of naturopathic medicine); hydrotherapy, physical therapies, including osteopathy or massage, counselling and lifestyle modification; herbal medicine, homeopathy, Traditional Chinese Medicine, touch therapies including massage, acupressure, shiatsu, and yoga.

So the whole approach with Naturopathy is totally holistic and covers many therapies and support techniques to aid good health and healing. Naturopaths use a variety of tests to assess the patients' health to build up a complete picture. This includes the iris test, which is said to indicate the state of internal organs; the sweat patch, which tests for mineral imbalances; a blood test.

Consulting a Practitioner

A naturopath works similarly to other therapists and will do a detailed questionnaire of your medical history and your lifestyle. The practitioner will then give you a routine medical examination, including tests on your blood pressure, lungs and heart, spinal joints and reflexes. The practitioner may also arrange for X rays, blood, urine and other tests.

A naturopath may diagnose your condition in terms unfamiliar to conventional doctors, such as 'toxic accumulation' and 'leaky gut'. Treatment falls into two broad categories. Catabolic (cleansing) treatment is given for conditions caused by a build up of waste products, and may include fasting to assist detoxification. Anabolic (strengthening) treatment is aimed at building up a weakened constitution with nutritional supplements and changes to diet. The practitioner may give advice about breathing patterns, exercise and relaxation. Some naturopaths are trained in counselling skills.

Advice is tailored to individual needs, and willing participation in treatment and a positive mental attitude are crucial. Your health should improve steadily, possibly with temporary relapses known as 'healing crisis' as detoxification takes effect.

As Naturopathy is totally holistic in its approach, I feel this therapy is extremely relevant to assist with healing for endometriosis. The techniques and support that are offered covers most areas of assistance needed, especially if the naturopath can offer counselling as well. Naturopathy is used a lot for conditions that are degenerative and long term, so Naturopaths will have relevant experience to deal with deep-rooted health problems such as endometriosis.

Success with Naturopathy

Catherine Nash, consultant, aged 32

'It is easy to feel a victim, not in the least because my GP couldn't help me with my endometriosis. It was making my life hell and my husband was at his last tether. Undaunted and in the profound belief that all illnesses can be cured I sought Naturopathic help.

I was given a new dietary regimen of no dairy, meat, or eggs, and no white refined products such as pasta, white bread, and white rice. No ready-made meals. I had to learn how to cook properly. We eat plenty of fresh organic vegetables and whole grains foods now. Yes my husband supported the diet change all the way. I was given herbs to cleanse and detox the body, particularly the liver, and to regulate my menstrual cycle. My Naturopath told me most gynaecological problems stem from liver imbalance.

My condition improved fabulously, which was very noticeable with each month. My overall health is now better than ever and completely clear of the former condition. I am so impressed I am taking up the study of Naturopathy to help others.'

With a few dietary and lifestyle changes, supplements, as well as herbal support, it can be managed very successfully. I myself have had endometriosis since I was 24. I had emergency surgery and hormone therapy, but later refused to have a hysterectomy! When I finally talked with Naturopathic doctors and Herbalists, I found out so much more about this condition, that none of the doctors I had seen were even aware of. I adjusted my diet, took an herbal combination for several months, and went from to severe pain, to completely normal, pain-free cycles ever since! It has been over 8 years now, and I have had NO return of symptoms! My periods are great, I am happy and doing what I love!'

* * *

'Apart from the pain, things went wrong when I was 20 - I bled for three months - non-stop. The doctor prescribed a high dosage contraceptive pill. The bleeding stopped but the pain continued. Eight years later Endo was diagnosed & Primulot prescribed. The pain went away (for a while) - that was wonderful. My mood improved out of sight - terrific! I gained weight which I could not shift - that was not wonderful. The pain returned and the weight stubbornly remained. Twelve years on, I found a Naturopath and Herbalist who makes individual prescriptions; over a few months, the pain went away (that was wonderful) - and my energy improved (bonus!).'

Ayurveda

The major traditional holistic healing system of the Indian subcontinent, Ayurveda covers all aspects of health, encouraging physical, mental, emotional, and spiritual well being. Practitioners believe well being is affected by three doshas, or 'vital energies', which constantly fluctuate. Treatment aims to restore health through purifying techniques, diet, yoga postures, and breathing exercises, massage, and herbal remedies. Therefore Ayurveda is very similar to Naturopathy.

Ayurveda (Sansrit for 'science of life) has been used on the Indian subcontinent since about 2500 B.C. It is a sophisticated health system, and has similarities with Traditional Chinese Medicine. For thousands of years Ayurveda was a well-regulated oral tradition. It remained the most accessible form of health care for Indians until the 19th century, when the British Raj attempted to stamp it out. Following Indian independence in 1947, Ayurveda underwent a revival. A central Council now monitors training and practise, with colleges offering a degree course that includes a basic study of Western medicine.

Ayurveda also works with the bodies' own life energy. Ayurveda teaches that there are five great elements - ether, air, fire, water, and earth - which underlie all living systems and are constantly changing and interacting. They can be simplified into three doshas, or vital energies. In the human body, the levels of the doshas are believed to rise and fall daily affected by factors such as different foods, time of day, season, level of stress, and repressed emotions.

Ayurveda places great importance on diet and detoxification techniques designed to purge the system by means of sweat, urine, and faeces. Herbal remedies, yoga, massage, and meditation are also believed to balance the system. Scientific studies of Ayurveda have shown the success of an herbal remedy being used, which contain antioxidants and was shown to reduce tumours in rats.

Consulting a Practitioner

At the first consultation the practitioner identifies your doshic constitution and any imbalances in it. They will ask detailed questions about your personal and family history and about your lifestyle. There are standard tests, examining the tongue, the pulse and the eyes.

The practitioner will recommend dietary changes to rebalance your doshas. They will advise you to eat at certain times of the day, depending on your age and condition. If your practitioner is qualified to prescribe medicinal remedies, they will also treat you with herbs and minerals. If you are considered strong enough, you may begin treatment with a cleansing and detoxification regime, which takes the form of enemas and laxatives. Saunas may also be used in preparation for detoxification.

Some practitioners offer Ayurvedic massage with oils. This lasts about an hour and is carried out by two masseurs, who work together on either side of you, stimulating your body's mama points (similar to acupoints), to encourage the flow of prana. Finally, the practitioner may suggest a rejuvenating regime that may include herbal remedies, yoga, meditation and sunbathing.

* * *

Choosing a Therapy

There are many complementary approaches to health, often with a confusing overlap of influences and theories, and an immense variety of methods for diagnosis and treatment. With the increasing popularity of complementary and alternative medicine, the number of therapies available has grown enormously.

The instincts you have about a therapy or a practitioner are important, as belief and trust play a significant role in healing. Make sure that your practitioner is reputable and well trained.

You are likely to respond better to a therapy if its principles fit with your ideas on well being and if you feel comfortable with its approach. Some of the things to consider about the type of therapy to use are:

- are you happy about being touched or having a massage
- are you OK about swallowing pills and can usually remember to take them regularly
- are you comfortable exploring your feelings with another person
- would you be prepared to change your diet radically
- can you tolerate the idea of having needles stuck in you
- are you comfortable about the practitioner manipulating your body
- do you mind getting undressed in front of the practitioner
- are you happy with the idea that you can use your mind to influence your health

Finding a Practitioner

Establishing a sense of rapport and trust with your practitioner is an important element of therapy if any benefits are to be derived from the treatment. Another key factor is of course, finding a competent practitioner.

Finding a good practitioner may be simply a matter of trial and error, and there are many people who prefer to rely on work-of-mouth recommendations. However, this approach is not necessarily reliable.

Training for alternative practitioners can range from as little as a correspondence course lasting only one weekend to three to four years of full or part time degree study.

Make sure that the therapist/practitioner you are considering is adequately trained and reputable. Before embarking on any course of therapy you should ask your practitioner these questions:

- What are the practitioners' qualifications? What sort of training was undertaken, and for how long?
- For how many years has the practitioner been in practise?
- Is the practitioner registered with a recognised professional organisation, and does that organisation have a public directory?
- Does the organisation have a code of practise, specifying the professional code of conduct?
- Is treatment available on referral by your doctor? Some therapies, such as chiropractic, osteopathy and acupuncture, are becoming accepted into mainstream medicine.
- Can you claim for the treatment through your health insurance, if you have it?
- What is the cost of treatment?
- How many treatments might you expect to require?

Trust and empathy are important with your practitioner, and treatment is unlikely to succeed without it. Treatment is often conducted on a one-to-one basis, so trust is imperative.

The Length and Effectiveness of Treatment

This depends on a number of factors including:

- the severity of the condition
- how long the person has been ill - as a general rule, however many years one has been ill, it takes as many months to recover
- the age and vitality of the patient, including hereditary factors. The younger the patient, the more vitality there should be
- the complications arising as a result of drug therapy
- how much effort the patient puts into treatment or how much the patient works against it
- the psychological attitude of the patient - whether she actually wants to get better
- the relationship between the patient and the practitioner

The Healing Crisis!

Finally, you need to be made aware and prepared for a fundamental piece of advice regarding the healing process, which any alternative health practitioner should give you - there is a phase of healing of the body called 'The Healing Crisis'. This is usually near the beginning of your healing. This is when the body is going into overdrive working hard to rebalance the system, get rid of unwanted toxins, and working to gear up the immune system. You will feel drained and tired and probably run-down.

This is going to make you feel worse for a short while, rather than better. This is a crucial time for your body to organise its healing capabilities, but it is also a time when many people give up on trying to heal naturally.

It stands to reason that this 'healing crisis' period will make you feel worse when you consider the amount of work your body is doing. This is why people feel so tired after an operation. The body is working very hard to heal from the trauma and repair the damage. It is the same when you have a virus or an infection, your body is working hard to suppress and destroy the invading infection.

If you continued to function as normal, you would be using vital energy that should be used by your body for healing, repairing damage, destroying germs and viruses. It is nature's way to make you sit down and STOP. Nature will knock you off your feet to make sure you can heal. This is why you do not heal when you take modern drug therapy for illness - you are not healing, you are masking the problem.

So be prepared to feel drained, and maybe worse than you do already. Just be reassured that this is a natural process. Do not start to worry that any alternative medication like herbs or homeopathic remedies is the cause of this feeling. These remedies will have kick-started your healing. With endometriosis there seem to be so many imbalances of the body to put right, and to enable real healing will involve a lot of restoring of many complex bodily systems

The length of time for this healing crisis will vary greatly from one person to another. It all depends on how seriously the body has become out of balance. It could be a few weeks, or anything up to a few months before you start to feel a shift in the right direction towards improvement. Just hang in there and be patient.

* * *

Lots of Self Help Stuff

The Power of Positive Emotions

Research shows there is a strong link between happiness, optimism, and good health and between increased well being, and the body's potential to heal itself. Exercises in positive thinking are beneficial, but more powerful still are positive emotions, such as hope and joy. Not surprisingly, close and supportive relationships with friends and family, and a sense of humour, can help to develop positive feelings.

A network of friends and family may be more important than we realise; a need to find emotional sustenance through others is a strong element in the pattern of healing and well being. The more isolated we are, the less healthy we are likely to be, since it can be difficult to have a rich emotional life alone. That is why it is so important for single women with endometriosis to foster and develop good relationships with their family and friends. Sometimes this can be difficult, for reasons I have discussed earlier, but the more you inform, advise and educate your friends and family, the more they will understand your needs. Some women with endometriosis have found huge support from their family, which has proved to be a lifeline for them spiritually and practically.

It is unfortunate that we do not all have loving, supportive families provided by our close relatives. In this case you need to look to other members of your family. Your Aunt or Grandmother may be more supportive than your mother or sisters. For that reason look further afield in your own family. My own Grandmother was very supportive. She could not do much practically as she lived miles away, but she was there to listen to me on the phone, and I could always write long candid letters to her which she replied to with supportive advice.

Do not become too distressed if some of your friends start to disappear. This is another subject I have already touched on. If your friends do start to fade away, then there will be a variety of reasons. Some people simply cannot face or cope with other peoples' illness. Then there is always the natural process that takes place in your relationships and people move on; your relationships change as you move through life. You will meet new people; make new friends, as you move in different circles in life.

If you start an evening course, for example, you may find yourself 'clicking' with certain individuals and you develop new friends. If you have a local Endometriosis Support Group in your area, then go along. You will make new friends. When I recovered from endometriosis and was fit and well again, I became involved in all sorts of activities, partly because I wanted to do the activity and partly because I knew it would bring me more rewards by meeting new people. Even if you are not feeling fit, vibrant and energetic, you could still take up new interests like join a yoga group, join a meditation group; join a poetry reading/writing group. There are lots of possibilities.

Do not hold yourself back through lack of self-esteem, and feelings that you are not interesting enough now, because your whole life seems to revolve around endometriosis. Your affirmative action to go out there and have a life is about you saying to yourself that your entire life is not about endometriosis. You do have a history, a background, a personality, personal interests; things you can give to others; things you can share with others. I say these words especially for those women who feel as though their life is closing in on them, (like it did for me in the beginning) and for those women who are suffering from very low self-esteem caused by endometriosis and all its consequences.

You need to break the vicious circle now, before it becomes self-perpetuating. Yes, you do have certain days when you feel too awful physically to do absolutely anything. BUT, make the most of the good days, and get out, get involved in your own life; do not let it pass you by because you think there is no point. There is every point. The point is, the more 'little' things you do, the more positive it will make you feel; and this will in turn assist you back to good health.

The value of relationships with regard to your health or recovery from illness should not be underestimated. A study at the University of California published in 1993 found that when patients with malignant melanoma had weekly support sessions that included education, stress management, coping skills, and discussion, they felt better and were more positive, although their defences showed little change. Six months later, when the support groups had discontinued, two-thirds of the group showed a rise in natural killer cell activity and enhanced immune system response. This was due to the sharing and supportive nature of being involved in the group, which had long-term beneficial effects.

Hope and humour are other important emotions to assist you in your well being and health. Hope is a component of optimism. It need not be unrealistic - in fact, hope can mean facing up to a problem and then looking for ways forward. Hope comes from having control of your life. Hopelessness comes from not having control in your life. Do not let endometriosis control your life. It is now time for you to take control of it. Just by reading these words is part of that process.

Having laughter and a sense of humour goes a long way to not only improve your life but also improve your health. Laughter eases muscle tension, deepens breathing, improves circulation, and releases endorphins, the body's natural pain-relieving opiates. It also raises levels of immunoglobulin A, an antibody in the mucous lining of the nasal cavity, and helps release hormonal substances called cytokines that promote the activity of 'natural killer' while blood cells. These cells specialise in fighting off invading bacteria and viruses, and in destroying potential tumour cells.

When you feel good about yourself you can accept your own imperfections. Being under stress and unable to cope, however, can undermine self-esteem and make you interpret every unfortunate event as the end of the world. Try to change the perspective by 'reframing the image' - you are not a failure if you do not succeed, but rather a success for trying. Even quite small shifts in self-perception can bring about profound changes in life.

Counselling

Counselling and psychotherapy covers a wide range of techniques used to ease psychological suffering. Whether treating mental and emotional disorders or promoting self-awareness, these therapies offer the chance to understand and resolve difficult thoughts, feelings and situations by talking to a skilled listener.

Counselling usually focuses on specific problems, such as bereavement or issues around illness, or job loss, rather than deep-seated personal issues. A counsellor is supportive and skilled in listening, and will prompt you to talk freely, but will probe less deeply than a psychotherapist, and will only offer limited advice. Instead, your thoughts and feelings are reflected back to you to increase your self-awareness. A counsellor will also help you to look at your situation from different perspectives in order to gain fresh insights and find your own solutions. If you are depressed or lack self-confidence, you may feel encouraged to stand up for yourself, or you may learn to express difficult emotions, such as anger, sadness or fear.

Seeing a counsellor can help you to obtain objective feedback about your own personal situation. Counselling gives you the space to explore your own thoughts and feelings. Sometimes, during these explorations, you may have a sudden insight into your own situation, which only by talking freely allows this to happen. Yes it is valuable to talk to friends, family, or your partner, but these people have a vested interest; they will not be able to listen objectively; they will have the tendency to interrupt you while you are in full flow, which can be quite destructive and deflating for you emotionally; also their own emotions will weigh in on the situation. Therefore it is the value of having someone who will really listen that is important in counselling. By expressing your needs, worries, anger, and all the other emotions, you are giving yourself the chance to vocalise and clarify what action to take.

There are so many people today who suffer from what I call 'Interrupitus'. These people will be engaged in a conversation with you, and as soon as you hit on a topic that hits home or has any relevance to them, then they go off on a complete rant of self-focussed dialogue, forgetting that this was your topic, and you wanted to air your views. Where have peoples listening skills gone these days? This is one of the problems facing women who suffer from endometriosis, in that other people seem to be extremely wrapped up in their own lives. This causes a huge hurdle for real honest communication to take place and women cannot talk freely about how they feel.

Dealing with endometriosis, is a huge burden on the emotions. This burden could prove too much not only for yourself, but also to pour out onto your loved ones. By seeing a counsellor, some of this burden can be lifted. It may also help you decide what action to take with regard to your treatment; what actions and decisions you need to take in life regarding things like work, finances and other practical issues in life.

When choosing a counsellor you need to ask about training and qualifications, and whether she (I feel it is advisable for you to see a female counsellor) belongs to a professional body. It is essential to trust your counsellor and that you feel relaxed with them. Otherwise the process will be counter-productive.

Meditation

Meditation is a mental discipline included in the practise of many world religions. Meditation is intended to induce a state of profound relaxation, inner harmony, and increased awareness. Various techniques can be used during meditation; all involve focusing the mind on a particular object or activity. This is why I enjoy African drumming so much, because it is an activity that totally focuses the mind on a single activity, and research has found that drumming induces the same alpha brain waves that are produced when meditating.

Several studies conducted by scientists have shown that meditation may induce profound change, far beyond the simple relaxation that most people use it for in the West, even beyond the medical applications of relieving stress, reducing blood pressure, and so on. In the late 1960s, Dr. Keith Wallace of the University of California found that the brain became more alert and the body more relaxed during meditation. Results from many other clinical studies include more orderly brain functioning, improved circulation of the fingers and toes, as well as reductions in anxiety, mild depression, insomnia, tension headaches, migraines, irritable bowel syndrome, and pre-menstrual syndrome.

Other research has found that regular meditators are biologically younger that those who do not meditate. In 1986, the Blue Cross-Blue Shield insurance did a study based on two thousand meditators in Iowa, which showed that they were much healthier than the American population as a whole. They studied seventeen major areas of serious disease, both mental and physical. The meditation group was hospitalised 87 per cent less often than non-meditators for heart disease and 50 percent less often for all kinds of tumours. There were equally impressive reductions in disorders of the respiratory system, the digestive tract, clinical depression, and so forth.

It is possible to teach yourself to meditate from books, tapes and videos, but you will probably find it easier to consult a teacher who will show you how to achieve a meditative state, as well as supervise your progress. Sessions may take place on a one-to-one basis or in groups. Practitioners use a variety of techniques, if you do not feel comfortable with one method then try another.

Whichever approach you choose, there are a few basic requirements for practising meditation successfully: a quiet environment where you can meditate without being disturbed, a comfortable position - usually sitting so as to prevent you from becoming drowsy or falling asleep, and a focus for the mind to help it withdraw form external reality. The object of meditation is a state of 'passive awareness', in which the mind is gently directed back to the focus of attention whenever it wanders, which it naturally does. Slow breathing and an awareness of the breath entering and leaving the body also help to promote deep relaxation. It is advised to meditate on a daily basis for around 15 - 20 minutes, preferably at the same time of day.

For women with endometriosis, meditation will be of benefit because it is said to aid with long-term pain, and enhances the immune system. This is an activity that will not cost you anything, especially if you are able teach yourself. There are often local meditation groups that meet, and people meditate together. This can help to focus the mind on the moment, if you are comfortable with working in a group. Some people prefer to meditate quietly alone because they feel less self-conscious and more relaxed. There are lots of meditation music tapes available, and these will help to cut out the background noise that we all suffer so much in modern life. These tapes consist of soft, quiet, relaxing music that is composed to last the entire side of the tape, so there are no sudden breaks.

Yoga

Yoga is a form of gentle exercise consisting of body postures and breathing techniques. It is a complete system of mental and physical training, originally developed as preparation for spiritual development. It has been practised for thousands of years in India as part of the Ayurveda system, and has now become popular around the world. In the West it is valued more for its physical than spiritual benefits, such as its ability to increase suppleness and vitality, and to relieve stress.

Today there are many types of yoga, including yoga therapy to maintain health and help specific medical conditions. While meditation is central to some forms of devotional yoga, the most popular form in the West is hatha yoga. Hatha means 'balance', reflecting the balance of mind and body. Yoga focuses on using specific postures of the body to bring about balance. These postures are called asanas. The other main focus is the use of breathing techniques called pranayama.

The yoga asanas and relaxation techniques were developed to bring physical and spiritual benefits. Hatha yoga has a physiological effect on muscle tone and circulation. Various asanas are believed to affect the autonomic nervous system and endocrine glands, which regulate internal functions, including heart rate and hormone production.

Most people find it helpful to join a beginners' class before continuing on their own. It is advisable to attend classes given by a qualified teacher. Most yoga classes last 40 - 90 minutes. After guiding you through gentle warm-up exercises, your yoga teacher will show you the correct way to perform yoga postures, which you will then be asked to practise with the other pupils in the class. Sitting and standing postures are held for between 20 seconds and 2 minutes and are designed to stretch and strengthen the body.

When practising yoga by yourself it is important to progress gradually and not to force your body into postures - especially for the more advance postures - before you are ready. Whether or not you are attending a yoga class, you should aim to practise for at least 20 - 30 minutes a day. Find a regular time, either before breakfast of before your evening meal. Regular daily practise should increase energy and stamina, tone muscles, improves digestion, enhance concentration, help you deal with stress better, and give you a greater sense of control.

The very gentle nature of yoga as a form of exercise is ideal for endometriosis sufferers. It allows the opportunity to take some form of exercise, which has many benefits, but is not too strenuous or taxing on the system. There are a few postures that are not advisable during pregnancy and, according to some experts, during menstruation. You can get advice from your yoga teacher about this.

Benefits of Yoga

- Stimulates glands and functioning of the immune system, enhances recovery from illnesses
- Reduces the effects of stress
- Improves focus, concentration and mood

- Alleviates insomnia
- Spiritual, intellectual and creative energies are released
- Counters obesity, assists in normalisation of weight
- Can support treatment of addictions and eating disorders

Cardiovascular Benefits
- Can normalise blood pressure
- Tones the muscles of the heart
- Can help to reduce cardiac disorders
- Improves circulation, minimises varicose veins

Musculoskeletal Benefits
- Lengthens the spine and improves its alignment
- Corrects bad posture
- Counters the effects of ageing on the spine and bones, tones muscles
- Prevents osteoporosis, builds bone
- Prevents hernia
- Prevents and treats back problems, including disc conditions; decompresses the spine
- Relieves sciatic and arthritis pain, can retard the progress of arthritis
- Keeps muscles flexibility and joints movable
- Corrects flat feet
- Relieves lower backache

Respiratory Benefits
- Improves breathing capacity
- Studies show improvement in asthmatic symptoms
- Can improve sinus conditions
- Increases the elasticity of lung tissue

Hormonal Benefits
- Normalises the menstrual cycle, checks heavy menstrual flow and relieves menstrual pain
- Helps to prevent hot flashes
- Can increase fertility

Digestive Benefits
- Rejuvenates abdominal organs and improves digestion
- Can improve haemorrhoids, constipation and flatulence
- Relieves stomach ache, reduces gastritis and acidity
- Helps calm irritable bowel syndrome, ulcers and colitis

Drug Free Ways to Manage your Pain

Nearly every woman who has endometriosis suffers from pain. This pain can be of varying degrees. It can also range from being continuous throughout the month, to being focused around the time of menstruation and ovulation. There are some women who, after a confirmed diagnosis of endometriosis, and have been found to have severe endometriosis, have had very little pain. Then there is the other end of the spectrum, of women with less invasive endometriosis, having severe crippling pain throughout the month.

Thus it is not totally clear what the physical/biological causes of endometriosis pain are in all cases, as it affects women in different ways. Many doctors do not understand the pain processes with endometriosis. There are some obvious sources, like the pain that will be caused by adhesions, inflammation and scarring. Endometriosis can also inflame the peritoneum, which is the membrane lining the abdominal cavity. This lining is similar in its structure to our skin, and sensory nerve endings, or receptors, are most highly concentrated in the skin. When stimulated by heavy pressure, extreme temperature, swelling or injury, they then send out the messages of pain. This is done by the chemical release of prostaglandins from the injured site, which relay messages to the brain. I am not going to speculate further about the various causes of pain; what I want to focus on here is how to manage it, rather than discuss it.

Our bodies have their own natural painkillers called endorphins. They slot into receptors located in the brain, spinal chord, and nerve endings, blocking pain impulses. How much information reaches pain receptors depends on the level of endorphins in circulation. This level is affected by our psychological state. Emotions can affect the perception of pain. Remember earlier I mentioned that laughter increases the amount of endorphins being released in the body; so the high you get from laughter will help reduce the sensations of pain, as the messages are being masked by extra endorphins being released. Likewise, pain may be perceived as being worse if the person experiencing it is depressed.

Conventional treatment for short-term pain is the prescribing of painkilling drugs ranging from aspirin to narcotics. Aspirin works by preventing the production of prostaglandins and reducing inflammation. Narcotics mimic endorphins, blocking pain impulses at specific sites.

Traditionally, drugs have been the primary means of controlling pain because they are simple, effective, and in most cases, safe. However, there are many people who are less tolerant of drugs and they may experience potentially harmful side effects, such as constipation, dizziness and nausea; and there may also be the risk of addiction.

T.E.N.S for Pain Relief

What is TENS?

Transcutaneous electrical nerve stimulation (TENS) is a drug-free method of pain relief that has been used to treat a wide variety of muscle and joint problems, as well as many other painful conditions. TENS uses electrical impulses to stimulate the nerve endings at or near the site of pain, diminishing the pain and replacing it with a tingling or massage-like sensation.

TENS can be used in a health-care setting, but most often people use it at home, by purchasing their own equipment. It is a safe, non-invasive, drug-free medically proven method of pain management.

How does TENS work?

Researchers still are not certain exactly how TENS works. The two explanations suggested most often are that electrical stimulation of the nerves blocks the pain sensation and that TENS trigger the release of the body's natural painkillers, called endorphins.

A TENS device consists of an adjustable power unit and electrodes that attach to the power unit via wires.

- The typical power unit is small — about the size of a beeper or a cell phone. Controls allow the patient to adjust the intensity of the stimulation. Some units also adjust for either high frequency or low-frequency stimulation. Frequency is a measure of the number of electromagnetic waves in a given time period.

- Electrodes come in a variety of shapes. They usually are self-adhesive and made of cloth or foam. A gel is applied under the electrode to improve the flow of current.

Before beginning treatment, you put the electrodes in place — usually on top of or next to the painful area. You can experiment with different locations for the electrodes to see what provides the best pain relief. In some cases, it may be more effective to position the electrodes on top of a related nerve or a site that is considered to be a trigger point or acupuncture point for the painful area.

Different types of TENS?

Electrical stimulation can be used in the following ways:

- **Conventional TENS** — This is the most typical type of treatment. It uses a high stimulation frequency, but the intensity of the electrical stimulus is low. People usually leave the electrodes on for long periods of time, turning them on and off at intervals. A typical treatment might last 30 minutes, but the length can vary depending on the persons needs.
- **Acupuncture-like TENS** — In this case, the stimulation frequency is low, but the electrical impulse is quite intense. Some people find this more effective or longer lasting than conventional TENS. Other people find acupuncture-like TENS too uncomfortable.
- **Percutaneous electrical nerve stimulation** — PENS, as it is known, is a combination of acupuncture and electrical stimulation. Instead of electrodes, PENS uses needles to penetrate the skin and deliver the electrical stimulation. This form of treatment would only take place under medical supervision.

How effective is TENS?

TENS has been used in patients with muscular pain, osteo-arthritis, rheumatoid arthritis, sciatica, and pain after surgery and other conditions.

Studies have shown varying results as to how well TENS works, what types of pain it can best relieve and how long the relief lasts. Many people have found TENS helpful, however, and it appears to work best for persistent pain. The equipment can be purchase on the Internet from a variety of suppliers, in Europe and the US. Prices do seem to vary, for example on US web sites they were priced from $150 to $300, so it will be worth shopping around.

Other Alternatives in Pain Relief

The symptoms of pain and its psychological effects can be helped by complementary approaches.

Massage

Studies have shown that massage can alleviate muscle pain and tissue-injury pain. The considerable psychological effects of massage may also be useful for persistent pain.

It may not be suitable to do regular deep muscular style massage on the abdomen to help with the pain of endometriosis. A more gentle approach may be needed. How many of you will naturally and unconsciously start rubbing your tummy when you have abdominal pains. It is a natural reaction because it is soothing. You do the same when you fall and hurt yourself; you immediately rub the area that has been injured or hurt, because it is like self-healing.

Try giving yourself a gentle abdominal massage using massage oil mixed with anti-spasmodic and healing essential oils.

The following oils are all anti-spasmodic:

Lavender, Thyme, Sage, Peppermint, Melissa

You could also use:

Rose - which is excellent for the reproductive system (but expensive)

Jasmine - excellent for uterine disorders

Aromatherapy

As well as using essential oils to massage the abdomen, as mentioned above, some essential oils are said to stimulate endorphin production and, when used with massage, to encourage relaxation. The stress and anxiety caused by long-term pain can cause the muscles to become tense. This may accentuate the perception of pain, creating a self-perpetuating downward spiral. So the use of aromatherapy can help to break the cycle caused by long-term pain.

Acupuncture

Acupuncture is said to work partly by stimulating the release of endorphins and prostaglandin-suppressing cortico-steroid hormones. The insertion of needles in appropriate acupoints may also help relieve anxiety and depression associated with persistent pain.

Acupuncture treatments for pain are thought to improve blood circulation in painful areas, promote local metabolism, and transform some pain inducing substances or strengthen analgesic substances in order to relieve pain. There have been control studies of the effectiveness of acupuncture for pain relief. Some studies have looked at the long-term benefits and have found that patients can still be pain free for up to 3 months after treatment.

Acupuncture and pain control

'Valerie is a 35-year-old single woman. She began to have unusual menstrual pain about five years ago when she was riding a bicycle while she had her period. Recently, her menstrual pain became severe, spreading to the vagina, anus, hips, and inner side of the thigh. A "sinking" sensation in the anus, with abdominal pain and back soreness accompanied the menstrual pain. Often, the pain was severe enough to trigger bouts of nausea and vomiting, and she became desperate for relief. She went to her regular doctor, who referred her to a gynaecologist. The pelvic examination, magnetic resonance imaging and laparoscopy confirmed that she had endometriosis. The gynaecologist suggested a hysterectomy, but she refused. She asked for other options. The doctor told her "acupuncture is effective to relieve pain. Why don't you try it?" She came to my clinic. After three month's treatment with acupuncture and Chinese herbal medicine, her endometriosis was under control.'

* * *

'It works! My endo pain during my period went from well above the pain scale of 10 to a 2. I have a life that I never had before. I don't understand completely how it works, but I would pay double *what I pay now (which is $120 a month) just to be able to live like I do. I tried everything from surgery to pain killers before and nothing works. If only I knew that such a non-invasive and totally safe procedure would work so well.'*

Yoga and Pain Management

Yoga is believed to reduce pain by helping the brain's pain centre regulate the gate-controlling mechanism located in the spinal cord and the secretion of natural painkillers in the body. Breathing exercises used in yoga can also reduce pain. Because muscles tend to relax when you exhale, lengthening the time of exhalation can help produce relaxation and reduce tension. Awareness of breathing helps to achieve calmer, slower respiration and aid in relaxation and pain management.

Yoga's inclusion of relaxation techniques and meditation can also help reduce pain. Part of the effectiveness of yoga in reducing pain is due to its focus on self-awareness. This self-awareness can have a protective effect and allow for early preventive action

Menastil

This is quite a new product to come on the market, which is produced for the relief of menstrual cramps. Menastil is the trade name for this product, which is receiving a lot of good feedback for the relief of pain associated with endometriosis.

Menastil is topically applied (applied to the skin), using a roll-on applicator. Many women have noted how fast and effective it is at relieving their pain and cramps. It is a homeopathic preparation and is available without prescription. The active ingredient is Calendula oil, which is effective as a topical analgesic and for pain relief.

Menastil has been clinically tested under strict FDA guidelines and found to provide safe, temporary relief from menstrual cramps. It has been tested on thousands of women over the past four years in double blind, placebo-based, cross over studies to test the efficacy of the product. Results of these studies showed that the vast majority of women tested found 'noticeable relief' to 'complete relief' after using it.

Menastil works by inhibiting the pain signals as they travel from one nerve cell to another. The junction, where these nerve cells connect with each other, is called a synapse. When applied topically, at the location of the pain, Menastil causes the endings of the nerve cells to retreat from each other and retract towards the cell body. This results in a reduction of the intensity of these impulses travelling to the brain and therefore a lessening in the amount of discomfort that is being registered by the brain.

Feedback on Menastil

The Endometriosis Research Centre received positive feedback on Menastil from women who participated in the initial focus study on the product. The following testimonials were part of the feedback the ERC received from women with endometriosis who have undergone repeated surgeries and are currently using pain management strategies ranging from acupuncture to narcotic pain relievers to cope with their symptomatic pain:"

"…took care of a good 80% to 90% of my cramps…smells wonderful and works like a charm. It lasts for about a week each time I use it."

'For mild cramps, it worked great; for hard cramps it takes the edge off. It has a pleasant smell [but strong smell]. For mild to moderate pain, I would rate it 6 to 8 on a scale of 1 to 10." I have always been

sceptical of trying anything new, especially when it claims to take away my cramps. However, when I was presented with an opportunity to try Menastil, an all-natural treatment, I thought 'why not?' Anything has to be better than taking pills to relieve the pain. Menastil took away the pain! Quick rub of the liquid on the spot of pain was all it took. Today, I woke up pain free; a huge difference from waking up with menstrual cramps that would sometimes have me doubled over in pain. In addition, the peppermint fragrance had a calming effect on me, and I believe it helped me get a better night's sleep."

"I used Menastil for pelvic adhesion pain. Within five minutes of application, the pain disappeared. It stayed gone for several hours and has not returned to that level since I used Menastil. Works fast and has no side effects whatsoever!"

"...After consulting with my massage therapist about trigger point therapy, I applied Menastil to the various trigger points that affect female organs. I achieved what I felt were greater results than that of just applying Menastil to 'problem areas.' Given my continuing determination for an all-natural approach to pain relief, I have been somewhat experimental with this product, but successful. I began using Menastil at the end of my menses, and what I found was it relieved nearly all of the frontal cramping and about 50% of the tailbone pain and leg cramps..."

These testimonials provide some hope for those women who suffer a lot pain associated with Endometriosis, and do not want to continue using painkillers because of the side effects. The product is natural, safe and generally effective. It is not particularly cheap, at around $40, but this is reported to last around 4 months on average. I have not seen any UK websites advertising this product, but it may be possible to get it shipped from the US.

DLPA

Endorphins are nature's painkillers. DL-Phenylealanine (DLPA) does not actually block the pain itself. It works instead by protecting the body's naturally produced pain killing endorphins (the body's morphine), effectively extending their life span in the nervous system. It slows the activity of "enzyme chewing" enzymes which destroy endorphins thereby giving them more time to act on areas of pain.

It helps the body to heal itself, and working through the brain, DLPA can also relieve some of the symptoms of other diseases. It is a powerful antidepressant and in clinical studies has been proven to be as effective as commonly prescribed antidepressant drugs - without the drugs' side effects. DLPA can also relieve symptoms of PMS and has had great success in dealing with the pain of endometriosis.

DLPA Dosage

Start with 375mg twice a day and then gradually increase to 2 x 375mg three times a day. Once this dose is reached, pain relief should start within a few days and should continue to bring relief for two to three weeks after the end of treatment. DLPA is non-addictive and you do not have to take larger or longer doses to reach the same effect. For some people a combination of DLPA and aspirin is beneficial. They work well together. Taking one coated aspirin (325 mg) in the morning helps to strengthen DLPA's effects. Also vitamin C and B6 appear to make DLPA more effective.

It takes anywhere from two days to three weeks for DLPA to take effect, so do not expect results straight away. Do not take DLPA if you are pregnant or breast-feeding and those with high blood pressure should take it after meals.

Arnica Gel and Cream

Arnica is a homeopathic remedy, taken internally and used for bruises, wounds, sprains, injury, as well as for tiredness after prolonged exertion. Arnica is also used in a skin preparation for the above, and is effective for pain relief. You could experiment with both.

Coping with Pain during Sexual Intercourse

Many women find that sexual intercourse is painful, both during and after intercourse. This situation simply compounds the guilt and adds more pressure to a relationship. It is estimated that about 60% of sufferers experience painful sex. There are certain practical things you can do to help this situation, for example:

- Make sure you are really fully aroused before penetration as it is less likely to cause pain, because you are properly lubricated. Full arousal also causes the vagina to elongate and the cervix to move further up and therefore you are less likely to hurt sensitive areas, such as the Pouch of Douglas or the pelvic organs.
- If you have problems with a dry vagina, try a natural lubricant such as vitamin E oil or Almond oil. There are products on the market for this purpose, but they do not feel very natural, whereas oils tend to feel nicer. It is quite safe to use these oils; the rule of thumb I use - never put anything on your body what you would not put inside your body.
- Try different positions for intercourse as this will alter the angle of penetration and in turn will alter the sensation of pressure inside your body to other areas
- Remember, that you do not always have to aim for penetration to enjoy a loving sexual relationship
- Make more special time for love making - have a warm bath together, light some candles, and try to get as relaxed as possible

Internal Support

Detox

Detoxification programmes will be valuable for endometriosis sufferers, because the process will off-load unwanted toxins that are in the system. Once these toxins have been eliminated then the body and the immune system can work better and will help to speed recovery.

Detoxification comes in many forms and refers to many different programs that cleanse the body of toxins. As mentioned earlier, our environment is toxic, the foods we eat contain many unwanted chemicals, and the air we breathe and the water we drink is laden with chemicals foreign to our system.

Detoxification for the body may refer to the cleansing of the bowels, kidneys, lungs, the liver or the blood, since these are the organs involved in detoxification of chemicals and toxins from the body. The liver acts as a filter for the removal of foreign substances and wastes from the blood. The kidneys filter waste from the blood into the urine, while the lungs remove volatile gases as we breathe.

Our body is designed to utilise natural substances for fuel, which includes foods, herbs and water. Any foreign substance will serve as a stimulus to our immune system, which has the function of removing these substances. Although the toxicity of a chemical may vary, it is the job of the liver to reduce toxins into compounds that the body can safely handle and eliminate through the kidneys (as urine), skin (as sweat), lungs (as expelled air) and bowels (as faeces). Maintaining these eliminative organs in good working order is essential for good health.

While there are many detoxification programs available, they differ in their actions and their intent. Some detoxification programs work only with the bowels, others may cleanse the liver or the blood, and others may aid the kidneys or the skin in their functions. By combining these detox programs into a total health program, you can effectively start to restore your health to an optimal level (and look younger in the process).

When the body can eliminate toxins, then health is restored and energy and vigour are revitalised. The process of detox can also aid and speed healing as the body will not be working so hard dealing with any toxic overload. Many different approaches to detoxification and wellness will work, even though they attack the problem at different levels. Other factors must be considered in detoxification, like nutrition, water intake, exercise, rest, sunshine, and fresh air.

Detoxification Diets

Detoxification diets help the body to eliminate toxins in many ways. First, natural vegetarian diets include the fibre needed for stimulating good bowel eliminate. They also contain the proper amounts of vitamins that feed and nourish the bowels and the liver, as well as other eliminative organs. They also include a valuable source of enzymes since many vegetarian diets include raw foods. The elimination of meat from the diet for a short period enhances detoxification because meat is difficult to digest and requires many enzymes for its digestion. Therefore, vegetarian diets are cleansing diets and aid the body in elimination of toxins.

For normally healthy people, detox diets will generally eliminate trigger foods, which may cause many problems with digestion and elimination. The foods to avoid while doing a detox are the foods which should be eliminated on a diet for endometriosis. (See further on for details)

Herbal Detoxification

In general diets for detoxification are good, but may not stimulate the liver, lungs or the kidneys as much as needed. Therefore, herbal cleanses are helpful when we want to cleanse more deeply and be organ specific. Herbs are powerful, because they may be combined together to fortify those herbs that aid specific organs.

While herbs may be taken at any time, they are best for detoxification purposes when they are used with a good diet. It does not make any sense to take herbs to cleanse the liver if the bowels are clogged with junk or refined foods, since the liver dumps its toxins into the bowels. And while detoxification diets are effective by themselves, they may be reinforced and speeded up with herbs, which stimulate the eliminative organs.

Herbs may be used as teas, powders or extracts. Powders are usually encapsulated for easier swallowing, but are best when taken with meals and digestive enzymes. Herbal teas are easily made and easily taken all throughout the day. They are mild and gentle and sometimes refreshing and sometimes bitter. Experimentation may be in order until you develop the right tea to drink.

To get the best advice about using herbs to aid a detox programme it may be a good idea to get advice from an herbalist or naturopath. Some herbs have estrogenic properties and getting guidance will help you avoid those herbs which are going to upset your hormone balance.

Skin Cleansing for Detox

Detoxification should include some type of skin cleansing, because our skin is one of our best eliminative organs. Heavy metals are actually released through the skin's pores when we sweat. Sauna baths and steam rooms are great for removing toxins from the skin and regenerating one's health and energy. It has been documented that our skin's sweat glands when combined can perform as much detoxification as one (or both) kidneys. Therefore, it is very important to support our skin for detoxification to be of maximum effect. If our kidneys are damaged, then helping the skin will help the kidneys ... indirectly, but effectively.

Also, good skin care is in order, if one's health is to benefit. Using chemical skin care products is not wise, even though they are cheaper. These chemicals are absorbed into our system and provide more "toxins" for our liver to deal with. The subject of toxic toiletries has briefly been covered in the previous chapter, but most people do not "see" the ill effects of these subtle chemicals, because their liver is able to metabolise them. But, individuals who are environmentally toxic will see a great change in their health when using natural soaps and shampoos.

Cleansing our skin is rather simple. First, we need to bathe daily using natural soaps. Then we need to care for the skin by using only natural oils and products of natural origin. Even the clothes we wear can make a big difference in our health. Synthetic fibres do not absorb sweat (toxins), while natural fibres, like cotton, will absorb toxins. Dry skin brushing helps in removing the outer dead skin layers and keeps the pores open. Another good method of skin brushing is with vigorous towelling off after bathing. Towel roughly until the skin is slightly red. Change towels often because they will contain toxins.

Detoxifying Baths

Use 1/2 cup of baking soda or use 1/2 cup of Epsom salt or use 1/2 cup of sea salt. Soak for 15-20 minutes and then scrub the skin gently with soap on a natural fibre. Within a few minutes the water will turn murky and "dirty." The darkness to the water is heavy metals coming out of the skin (aluminium and mercury). Do this once a week during detox and once a month for maintenance.

Juice Detoxing

Detoxing with vegetable and fruit juices can be another excellent way to develop good health and cleanse the body of toxins. The vitamins, minerals and enzymes of raw juices are absorbed into the bloodstream and get to work on the body within minutes. Detoxing on a juice diet and not eating any other foods will have the same benefits of doing a food fast. (See further on for details about fasting.)

When the pulp is not included, you are able to drink more juice than you would be able to eat of the same amount of un-juiced foods. For example, one can easily consume the juice of several heads of lettuce in one sitting, but may not be able to eat the lettuce whole. This allows the body to get an abundance of nutrients with minimal processing (digestion). Fasting on mono-juices also allows the body proper time to process these juices and helps to preserve our valuable digestive enzymes.

Juice fasting has helped many people over come serious diseases like cancer, because it gave them optimal nutrition and allowed the body to cleanse itself of toxins. [According to many nutritionists, cancer is merely a toxic condition.] With some juicers, the pulp is discarded, but it may be saved and added back for fibre (not too much). Juices contain good sources of antioxidants and enzymes, both of which are needed for cleansing and eliminating toxins. Juices are also easy to digest and help those with digestive problems. To get the same amount of nutrients as one gets from a pint of raw juice, one would have to eat plates of raw food. Raw juices have been used in many therapies to treat various illnesses.

To extract the juices from fruit and vegetables you need to buy a special juice extractor. These are different from electric blenders and food processors. They separate the juice from the pulp, either by direct pressure or centrifugal force. The most efficient type is the centrifugal one, which will extract much more juice.

There are various books available giving advice, ideas and tips of how to prepare fresh raw juices. Try your local library in the first instance.

Intestinal Flora and Detox

Our bowel flora is also important for detoxification and normal health. Probiotics is the term given to the normal bowel flora, which can be taken as supplements to re-balance the flora of your system. It has been found that these normal flora actually defend our body from the pathogenic species of bacteria and perform many vital functions, such as detoxification of toxic chemicals and making valuable vitamins (mainly the B vitamins). When our normal flora is present they secrete mediators in which the pathogenic forms cannot grow. But the reverse is also true, that when the pathogenic forms take over, they will exclude the normal flora with their toxins.

Antibiotics kill off the good bacteria as well as the bad and allow the bad to repopulate and develop antibiotic resistance. Natural forms of antibiotics are better, since they do not kill off the good bacteria with the bad, and do not allow drug" resistance to take place. Garlic, for example, is perhaps, 200 times more effective against pathogens than most antibiotics today. And it does not produce antibiotic resistance forms, which is a danger to all our health. As antibiotics become more widely used, more antibiotic resistant forms will be encountered. Herbal antiseptics and anti-bacterial tonics are far better and less dangerous to our over-all health, because they do not kill of the good bacteria with the bad.

Replacing our natural flora is a good step for preventing disease and keeping our bowels healthy and populated with normal flora. Taking probiotic containing Lactobacillus acidophilus and Bifidus can help us in our detox program and also in repopulating the gut after a cleanse. Our normal healthy flora should be a part of any detoxification program.

Antioxidants and Detox

The use of antioxidants, like vitamins A, E, and especially C, are very essential for detoxification since they are involved with the assimilation of toxins. Antioxidants are involved with helping cells to neutralise free radicals that can cause mutations and cellular damage. As these free radicals are neutralised, the antioxidant vitamins will be used. Vitamin A and E are fat soluble and will be found in our fat tissues/stores, but vitamin C is water soluble and will be found mainly in our skin.

Vitamin C is also involved with many other important bodily functions, like collagen formation, wound healing, and energy production and fighting off colds (viruses). The function of antioxidants is so important that any deficiency of them will be seen as catastrophic to one's health. When our antioxidants are low, energy is not available and detoxification cannot take place in a normal fashion. Therefore, toxins accumulate or are stored until they can be processed. The liver and many other organs are compromised in their functions when antioxidants are low. Just the lack of energy is enough to cause the body to have compromised or poor health, because it is energy that is required for the removal of toxins and wastes.

Vitamin C should be taken with bioflavinoids to ensure that all the components of the vitamin C complex are taken together, since they work together. Pure ascorbic acid is called vitamin C, but does little by itself. We tend to think that ascorbic acid as vitamin C, but it is only part of the vitamin C complex. Vitamin C is very essential to any detoxification program, because that is what the body uses for energy to process and eliminate these toxic wastes. Vitamin C can be taken in very high doses until the bowel tolerance level [BTL] is achieved. This BTL is different for different people. Some people reach tolerance at 4-5 grams (4,000-5,000 mg), while others may not reach tolerance until 10-15 grams (10,000-15,000 mg). Cancer patients can take 20-30 grams (20,000-30,000 mg) of vitamin C before tolerance is reached ... meaning that they needed more vitamin C than most people.

Enzymes

The use of enzymes in detoxification is important, because the body needs an adequate supply of enzymes, not only for digestion, for also for detoxification. Enzymes are best obtained from fresh raw fruits and vegetables, but may be taken daily with meals as nutritional supplements of multi-digestive enzymes. Enzymes in our food helps us to digest that food, but many foods today are processed, refined, heated (cooked), radiated and stored, which destroys enzymes and leaves it non-vital. Foods with enzymes destroyed will have a longer shelf life, but will not give you health benefits when it is eaten.

Fresh raw fruits and vegetables are the best source for enzymes and help to give you vibrant health. Enzymes are also used by the body in detoxification of toxic substances. The liver is the source of most detoxification enzymes, which it must make, or store. To aid the body in removing and eliminating wastes and toxins, enzymes are best taken in between meals. This way they do not get involved with digestion, but go to the liver and to the blood for detoxification.

Enzymes also help the bowels in cleansing, because they liquefy the bowel content, which makes transit much easier. The role of enzymes in digestion is to break down foods for digestion and absorption. When foods are broken down they become more liquid and the bowels move much easier and faster. Transit time is decreased and our health is increased when toxins are removed and eliminated. This is probably the link to breaking the "constipation chain" which many people in the West suffer from. Enzymes are the key to health.

Bowel Cleansing

Keeping the bowels clean and moving is a major step in regaining our health since the bowels are crucial in the elimination of toxins, especially those processed by the liver. (The liver dumps in to the bowel via the gall bladder.) This is why one hears a lot about the bowels, and bowel cleansing. In severe cases, enemas and colonics may be needed to break-up and washout long-standing bowel encrustations. Diet may do the same thing as an enema or colonic, it will just take longer. Also, one should be very diligent in repopulating after a total washout of the normal flora, and supplements of probiotics will be necessary to restore the balance in your system.

The easiest way to get the bowels moving is by using a high fibre diet consisting of fresh fruits and vegetables. Sometimes, you can add extra fibre during the day by drinking a glass of water or juice with psyllium husk powder. The extra fibre adds to the bulk of the stool and decreases the bowel transit time, which means better toxin elimination and better health. It makes sense that if you can eliminate toxins your health will improve.

To Sum up on Detox

A reaction can occur when the body is detoxifying and toxins are being released faster than the body can eliminate them. When this occurs, you can suffer from headaches, nausea, and general feeling of being run-down. This reaction should not last long, and the more you detox, the lighter the load is on the body.

To minimise any reaction:

- Drinks lots of pure water
- Get minimal exercise daily
- Lots of sunshine
- Take detoxification slowly... one step at a time
- Keep the organs of elimination (bowels, lungs, skin, kidneys) open
- Take detox baths
- Use aromatherapy oils for aches - like peppermint, birch, and wintergreen
- Sweat by using exercise, saunas, baths, and herbs
- Avoid foreign chemicals and refined processed foods

Detoxification is essential for good health to exist. Our body must eliminate toxins daily or we would die immediately. We have the added burden of toxins in our environment, as well as the natural toxins that we would find in our bodies anyway. Therefore there is a need to boost and assist the detoxification process of our bodies. Detoxification is a lifestyle change. It is the way we live that determines our health, and how we treat our bodies and what we put in them that maintain long-term health.

Candida Albicans

Many women have had great success in dealing with their endometriosis by following a diet regime that is designed to deal with Candida Albicans. There is much speculation that there is a link between Candida and endometriosis. The foods that should be eliminated in a diet for Candida are very similar to the foods that should be eliminated to deal with endometriosis. There are a few variations but the basics are the same.

For Candida, avoiding all forms of yeast forming foods, fermented foods, and mould foods is essential, as these will all help to feed the Candida yeast over-population. Candida albicans yeast normally lives harmlessly in the gastrointestinal tract and genito-urinary areas of the body. But, Candida may infect virtually any part of the body. The most commonly involved sites include the nail beds, skin folds, feet, mouth, sinuses, ear canal, belly button, oesophagus, intestine, vaginal tract and urethra. Candida also infects deep internal organs, which sometimes results in serious disease. Likely sites of infection include the thyroid and adrenal glands, kidneys, bladder, bowel, oesophagus, uterus, lungs and bone marrow.

In the past, Candida infection was regarded as a woman's problem because of its connection to a vaginal yeast infection. Today, we know that both men and women are equally likely to develop Candida. Candidiasis is really a state of inner imbalance, not a germ or bug. When immunity and resistance are low, the body loses its intestinal balance and Candida yeasts multiply too rapidly, voraciously feeding on sugars and carbohydrates in the digestive tract. It's an immune-compromised condition. Unless the body's weakened defences are given assistance, Candida colonies will flourish throughout the body and keep releasing toxins into the bloodstream.

Lifestyle factors that promote Candida infection

- Poor diet - especially excessive intake of sugar, starchy foods, yeasted breads and chemicalised foods.
- Repeated use of antibiotics - long-term use of antibiotics kill protective bacteria (that keep Candida under control).
- Hormone medications like corticosteroid drugs and birth control pills.
- A high stress life, too much alcohol, too little rest.

Some symptoms of Candida

- recurrent digestive problems, gas, bloating or flatulence
- rectal itching, or chronic constipation alternating to diarrhoea
- a white coating on your tongue (thrush)
- unusually irritable or depressed, unexplained frequent headaches, muscle aches and joint pain
- feel sick all over, yet the cause cannot be found.
- chronic vaginal yeast infections or frequent bladder infections
- psoriasis, eczema or chronic dermatitis
- catch frequent colds that take many weeks to go away
- oversensitive to chemicals, tobacco, perfume or insecticides. Crave sugar, bread or alcoholic beverages

Fasting

Fasting for short periods of time is the quickest way to detox the system. It is wonderfully effective in emergencies and works well to accelerate the healing of long-term illnesses. It can help to rebalance you mentally, physically, spiritually and emotionally.

The theory behind fasting is that the body comes well equipped with mechanisms for incinerating and eliminating nutritional waste as well as the toxic effects of stress, grief and anger. The digestive process uses up 30 per cent of the total body energy, so if the digestive system is placed in a complete state of rest, it can concentrate on detoxification and healing.

Fasting is also invaluable preventative medicine. Not only does it help the body to maintain peak fitness by periodically unburdening itself of accumulated waste, but it nips minor health problems in the bud, decelerates the ageing process, if done regularly stabilises body weight, and helps to prepare the body to utilise nutrition for more effectively after the fast is broken.

The Process of Fasting

Our bodies are continuously replacing our cells. Only by speedy and efficient elimination of the dead cells can the building and growth of fresh cells be stimulated. Fasting actually accelerates the elimination of dead cells and speeds up the building of new healthy cells. The cleansing capacity of all the eliminative organs of the body is vastly increased. For instance, the concentration of discarded toxins in the urine can be increased by up to ten times, and an over-burdened liver can dump its waste six times more quickly than usual.

How to Fast

You do not fast on water alone, particularly if you have never fasted before. It is a miserable experience for our bodies which would groan with toxins and the particularly potent one; the result of ingesting insecticides and poisonous metals, which would pour into the system so rapidly that you will finish up almost drowning in your own poison! It is better to choose either one type of fruit or alkaline juices.

Some people say that eating fruit is not a pure fast and it is true that the digestive organs are not allowed to rest as much as if only liquids were being processed. But eating fruit certainly ensures the incineration of old tissues, which is the requirement of fasting. Fruit fasting is good for first timers, and is especially good for dealing with constipation.

Most people make the mistake of not eating enough fruit and the secret to successful fasting is to eat as much of your chosen fruit as you can without being ridiculous about it. You need to aim for about 4 to 6 pounds of fruit per day, eaten at 2 hour intervals and let your digestion rest in between. Do not drink anything with your fruit, as this will dilute the digestive enzymes and make the fruit a less potential healing tool. You may drink as much mineral water between the fruit as desired.

If you enjoyed a few fruit fasts you can then go onto juice fasts, which are particularly beneficial, because you can ingest so much more in terms of quantity and therefore absorb more vitamins, trace elements, minerals and enzymes. You need to drink 30 ml of juice for every pound of your body weight. If that is impossible, dilute the juice to half and half with mineral water. You may well be drinking a gallon of liquid a day. The more liquid you take in, the quicker you flush out all the accumulated toxins and the less possibility there is of retaining water, because mineral water and juices act as natural diuretics.

If possible juices should be raw and freshly pressed from well-washed fruit. The most effective juicing machines are those that spin juices out by centrifugal action and operate continuously. These machines can be rather expensive, but I managed to obtain one by applying to a trust fund for a small grant. You do not have to stick to the same fruit throughout, but do have just one type of fruit in a given day.

If you have been taking medication, you should **not** stop taking it while fasting. You may have to reduce it to only a third or a quarter of the normal dose because it will take effect much more efficiently in the system. You should be getting all the vitamins and minerals you need from the goodness supplied in the fruit, so there is no need for supplements.

If you have never fasted before, try fasting for just one day a week for several weeks. Then go onto a three or four day fast, which is when you will begin to get the most benefit of off-loading the toxins in your system and be able to do some deep cleansing. Two day fasts are not as effective, as the liver is starting to build up to dumping toxins, but never quite gets there on the two-day programme.

Always choose a quiet time in your life to do a fast. Do not do one if you are depressed. Try not to watch television, and be selective of what you read. Go for gentle walks and get some fresh air. To break your fast, eat very lightly the first day; a piece of fruit for breakfast, a light simple salad for mid-day, and a light soup made from grains in the evening.

Controlled Diet for Endometriosis

The role of a controlled diet in endometriosis management has proved exceedingly beneficial for many women. The plan of the endometriosis diet is to relieve or prevent some of the disabling symptoms that occur with menstruation, as well as the general pain of endometriosis. The goal is to decrease estrogen levels, stabilise hormones, increase energy, alleviate painful cramps and stabilise emotions.

Endometriosis is an estrogen-sensitive condition, but the painful menstrual cramping that occurs is predominantly due to prostaglandin synthesis in the body. Prostaglandins are naturally occurring fatty acids, which are derived from dietary sources. The body can produce different types of prostaglandins through a complex series of pathways.

There are the 'good guys' and the 'bad guys' of the prostaglandin group. The goal of a controlled diet is to block the 'bad guys' (PGF2a and PGE2) for their negative actions on the body and increase the 'good guys' (PGE1) for their opposite and beneficial actions. The action of the bad guys is to increase uterine contractions, and the good guys have a soothing effect. By changing the types of oils that are taken into the diet, the production of the good guys can be stimulated, which helps with uterine relaxation. These oils are composed of omega-3 acids, which lead to PGE1 production. Excellent sources of the omega-3 fatty acid producing oils are:

- evening primrose
- Safflower oil
- Walnut oil
- flax seeds/oil

It is also important to decrease intake of those fatty acids that will stimulate the bad guys which are found in: saturated fats, butter, animal and organ meat, lard.

In addition to decreasing bad fat intake, the diet should also consist of high fibre. Not only does this help with good digestion, but it is also thought that a diet high in fibre can decrease total circulating estrogens. It is recommended to incorporate 25 grams per day of fibre. Good sources are:

- whole grains **excluding** wheat and rye
- beans, peas and pulses
- brown rice
- vegetable and fruits
- oatmeal

The following vegetables are recommended to modulate estrogen levels by incorporating one or two servings a day:

- kale
- collard greens
- mustard greens
- broccoli
- cabbage
- turnips

Foods to Avoid

- refined and concentrated carbohydrates
- sugar, in whatever form, including honey
- alcohol
- caffeine which is found in tea, coffee, soft drinks
- chocolate
- dairy produce including all milk and cheese
- fried food, margarine and hydrogenated fats
- soy based foods and products. Tofu and miso allowed in small amounts
- tinned and frozen packaged foods
- manufactured meat products

- additives and preservatives

Foods Beneficial for the Immune System
- beans, peas, lentils
- onions
- garlic (raw or lightly cooked)
- carrots (contain beta-carotene)
- live yoghurt (good for health intestinal flora)
- rhubarb
- seeds and sprouted seeds
- ginger
- green tea

Hormone Balancing Foods
Foods containing natural plants sterols can be helpful. They are thought to block the estrogen receptors, but are too weak to exert a very strong hormonal effect. These include:
- peas, beans and pulses
- red and purple berries
- garlic
- apples
- parsley
- fennel
- brassicas: cabbage, cauliflower etc.
- nuts and seeds
- celery, carrots
- rhubarb
- sage

To Sum Up
- increase omega-3 fatty acids
- decrease, or better still, avoid meat and dairy
- increase fibre
- modulate estrogen
- avoid sugars, caffeine and alcohol
- avoid refined foods, e-numbers, additives
- minimise or avoid soy products as they contain toxins, phytic acid and high levels of phytoestrogens (see more on this below)
- eat organic produce wherever possible
- drink lots of filtered or mineral water

Feedback sent to Endo Resolved
'The best thing that ever happened to me was being diagnosed with endo last year! Since 16 I had had difficult painful periods (which I thought was normal because of my mum's terrible problems) and the pain was sort of controlled by the Pill. After having 2 children in my early 30s, for about 8 years I had no period pain. Approaching 40 I started getting migraines, bad skin, irritable bowel syndrome, constant thrush, dreadful mood swings and weight gain. Taking supplements helped, but then when the period pain began a year ago, it was unbearable. I was diagnosed about July 06, and a hysterectomy sounded really good. I did my homework, thanks to endo-resolved, and

started the diet, cold turkey. I also increased my exercise regime. After 8 weeks I had lost 8 kilos, my skin cleared up, I had boundless energy and much less period pain. I decided on a laparoscopy & mirena. The specialist said I was making a mistake and would be back for the hysterectomy. After 6 months I have lost 15 kg, all of my symptoms are gone, I have no pain, and today for the first time in 30 years, my optometrist tells me my eyesight has improved - dramatically - which he can't explain. I have shared the diet with many friends and acquaintances, and some of them are starting to try it. Thanks for your help, it's literally changed my life.' S.D. New Zealand

Coconut Oil in your Diet

Coconut oil should be a serious consideration in your diet. The health benefits of Coconut oil appear to be far reaching, and some members of the press are calling this a 'wonder food'. The ability of Coconut oil to boost the immune system, as well as soothe and repair digestive disorders will be very relevant and supportive when you have endometriosis.

Coconut oil is now deemed as one of the healthiest oils you can consume. It is rich in lauric acid, which is known for being antiviral, antibacterial and antifungal. You can even use it on your skin to help prevent wrinkles.

In addition to tasting and smelling great, the health benefits of Coconut oil include:

- Help you lose weight as it speeds up the metabolism
- Reduce your risk of heart disease
- Lower your cholesterol
- Improve conditions in those with diabetes and chronic fatigue
- Improve Crohn's, IBS, and other digestive disorders
- Prevent other disease and routine illness with its powerful antibacterial, antiviral and antifungal agents
- Increase metabolism and promote healthy thyroid function
- Boost your daily energy
- Rejuvenate your skin and prevent wrinkles

There is a widespread misconception that coconut oil is bad for you because it contains saturated fat. Fats are categorised as short, medium, or long-chain depending on how many carbon molecules they contain. Close to two-thirds of the saturated fat in coconut oil is made up of medium-chain fatty acids, which have anti-microbial properties, are easily digested by the body for quick energy, and are beneficial to the immune system. Far from being dangerous, the saturated fat in coconut oil is actually health promoting.

Quality of Oil

You need be absolutely certain, however, of the quality and effectiveness of whatever coconut oil brand you choose. There is a very wide variety in terms of the types of coconuts, and the manufacturing processes used to make the oil.

Most commercial coconut oils are RBD (refined, bleached, and deodorised). RBD oils do contain the medium chain fatty acids, however they also contain chemicals used in processing. You need to purchase cold-pressed, virgin coconut oil - the same as you would for olive oil - to get the health benefits without the added chemicals.

How it works

Coconut oil's saturated fat is of the medium-chain fatty acid (MCFA) variety. These MCFAs are digested more easily and utilised differently by the body than other fats. Whereas other fats are stored in the body's cells, the MCFAs in coconut oil are sent directly to the liver where they are immediately converted into energy. So when you eat coconut oil, the body uses it immediately to make energy rather than store it as body fat. Because this quick and easy absorption puts less strain on the pancreas, liver and digestive system, coconut oil "heats up" the metabolic system and is outstanding for those with thyroid problems.

For those with Crohn's and IBS, the anti-inflammatory and healing effects of coconut oil have been shown to play a role in soothing inflammation and healing injury in the digestive tract. Interestingly, researchers have demonstrated the benefits of coconut oil on patients with digestive problems, including, Crohn's disease since the 1980s. Its anti-microbial properties also promote intestinal health by killing troublesome micro-organisms that may cause chronic inflammation.

Coconut oil supports the immune system by ridding the body of harmful micro-organisms, thus relieving stress on the body. With fewer harmful organisms taxing the body's energy, the immune system can function better.

For women with endometriosis, this oil can be incorporated into your diet in many ways - as cooking oil, added to salads in a dressing, as a spread in place of butter, or added to your baking. And don't forget that you can use it straight on your skin as a moisturiser.

Green Tea

There are many health benefits to be gained by consuming Green Tea. There is one health benefit in particular which will be very appropriate for women with endometriosis, and that is the ability of Green Tea to protect the body at a molecular level from the toxic effects of Dioxins.

The fact that researchers have discovered that Green Tea can protect the body from the damaging effects of dioxins is valuable advice for women with endometriosis, given that many researchers feel that dioxins could be the cause of endometriosis.

Green tea is actually the same plant as its more well-known cousin black tea; however, special processing retains a far greater antioxidant profile in green tea leaves, resulting in a far more superior beverage for supporting health. Numerous scientific studies now document the tremendous benefits of drinking green tea.

A study by researchers at Rochester University suggesting that green tea's ability to fight cancer is even more potent and varied than scientists had initially known about. The researchers found chemicals in green tea that shut down a key molecule that can play a role in the development of cancer. The molecule - the aryl hydrocarbon receptor, or AH - can activate genes in a harmful way. Dioxins and tobacco smoke cause the molecule to trigger potentially harmful gene activity. Two chemicals in green tea - similar to the anti-cancer flavonoids in cabbage, broccoli, grapes, and red wine - inhibit AH activity.

There are numerous chemical contaminants which enter the body and cause their damaging effects through the molecular pathway. This same pathway is shut down by the active ingredients in Green Tea. These chemicals include dioxins, some PCBs, and some polycyclic aromatic hydrocarbons among others.

Some of the numerous health benefits of green tea

Anti-aging, Cancer fighting properties - Studies have shown that, taken in sufficient quantities, green tea can:

- Block angiostatis, the new blood vessels tumours need to grow.
- Inhibit metastasis, the process by which cancer spreads in the body
- Reduce the production of DHT, a potent form of testosterone implicated in causing prostate cancer
- Lower in incidence of lymph node metastasis in post menopausal women
- Inhibit the onset of breast and colon cancer, as well as melanoma.
- Enhances the effectiveness of chemotherapy in ovarian cancer.
- Help protect DNA from radiation induced damage
- Can produce apoptosis (programmed cell death) in lung cancer patients, as well as protecting smokers from the onset of lung cancer.
- Prevent inflammation and possible subsequent skin cancer when applied to the skin.
- Can lower serum glucose and consequent insulin, reducing the possibility of tumours and immunosuppressive hormones.

Cardio-protective Qualities

The use of adequate amounts of green tea can:

- Increases the healthy function of the liver and pancreas
- Lower LDL cholesterol levels
- Lowers intestinal fat absorption
- May act as natural calcium-channel blockers
- Lower blood pressure because of its powerful vasodilatation properties
- Protect the brain from oxidative stress
- Raise the serotonin and dopamine levels in the brain
- Diminish the incidence of iron induced epileptic seizures
- Improve kidney function
- Protect the body from the ravages of oxidised linoleic acid produced by heating margarine, corn and safflower oils.
- Inhibit HIV virus replication
- Promote dental health by inhibiting the growth of unwanted oral bacteria.
- Destroy harmful intestinal bacteria and lowers the pH

Green tea provides powerful antioxidant polyphenols (estimated as 25X the antioxidant activity of vitamin E and 100X that of vitamin C). It promotes growth of friendly intestinal bacteria and decreases toxic bowel metabolites. Finally, another key benefit is the ability to greatly boost the immune system.

Drink Decaffeinated Green Tea

It is well known that caffeine aggravates the symptoms of endometriosis, but fortunately you can purchase decaffeinated Green Tea.

An average cup (6 oz) of green tea contains approximately 30 milligrams of caffeine. This compares to a cup of black tea, which has about 40 milligrams, and a cup of brewed coffee, which has 120 milligrams of caffeine. A cup of naturally **decaffeinated** green tea contains only 2 milligrams of caffeine per cup, so this will be safe to drink.

The effect of the decaffeination process on the health benefits of green tea depends on the decaffeination process. A natural decaffeination process preserves the antioxidants found in green tea by using only spring water and effervescence (CO_2 method) to take the caffeine out. Some Green Tea brands use the chemical, ethyl acetate, which can destroy most of the best antioxidants found in green tea. A double negative of more unwanted chemicals plus the health benefits of the tea being removed. Therefore if you want to give Green Tea a try then purchase naturally decaffeinated organic Green Tea, which will not upset or aggravate your symptoms of endometriosis.

A Word about Soy

In recent years soy has emerged as a 'near perfect' food, with supporters claiming it can provide an ideal source of protein, lower cholesterol, protect against cancer and heart disease, reduce menopause symptoms, and prevent osteoporosis, among other things.

Two isoflavones found in soy, genistein and daidzen, the same two promoted by the industry for everything from menopause relief to cancer protection, were said to 'demonstrate toxicity in estrogen sensitive tissues and in the thyroid'.

There are two 'camps' for the use of soy in food. There is the traditional, oriental use of soy in fermented soy products. These products are produced naturally and do not contain the same chemicals and toxins of the modern highly processed use of soy.

The modern approach to the use of soy has come by default, by finding a use of the soy bean by-products after the extraction of oil from the bean. There was so much soy bean residue that extensive multi-million dollar campaigning and advertising was used to promote this new 'wonder-protein'.

The soybean did not serve as a food in China until the discovery of fermentation techniques, some time during the Chou Dynasty. The first soy foods were fermented products like tempeh, natto, miso and soy sauce.

At a later date, possibly in the 2nd century BC, Chinese scientists discovered that a purée of cooked soybeans could be precipitated with calcium sulphate or magnesium sulphate (plaster of Paris or Epsom salts) to make a smooth, pale curd - tofu or bean curd. The use of fermented and precipitated soy products soon spread to other parts of the Orient, notably Japan and Indonesia.

The Chinese did not eat unfermented soybeans as they did other legumes such as lentils because the soy bean contains large quantities of natural toxins or "anti-nutrients".

Production of modern soy protein products takes place in industrial factories where a slurry of soy beans is first mixed with an alkaline solution to remove fibre, then precipitated and separated using an acid wash and, finally, neutralised in an alkaline solution.

Acid washing in aluminium tanks leaches high levels of aluminium into the final product. The resulting curds are spray-dried at high temperatures to produce a high-protein powder. A final indignity to the original soybean is high-temperature, high-pressure extrusion processing of soy protein isolate to produce textured vegetable protein (TVP).

But high-temperature processing has the unfortunate side-effect of so denaturing the other proteins in soy that they are rendered largely ineffective. Nitrites, which are potent carcinogens, are formed during spray-drying, and a toxin called lysinoalanine is formed during alkaline processing. Numerous artificial flavourings, particularly MSG, are added to soy protein isolate and textured vegetable protein products to mask their strong "beany" taste and to impart the flavour of meat.

Soy is found in dozens and dozens of items: granola, vegetarian chilli, a vast sundry of imitation animal foods, pasta, most protein powders and "power" bars, soy milk, soy yoghurts, soy based cheeses, to name just a few.

After multi-million dollar figures spent on advertising and intense lobbying to the Food and Drug Administration (FDA), about 74 percent of U.S. consumers now believe soy products are healthy. Here is a quote about soy from the book "What Your Doctor May Not Tell You About Pre-menopause" by Dr. John Lee, one of the pioneers in the use of Natural Progesterone Cream.

"Please be wary of all the hype around soy. Although it does contain compounds that can help balance your hormones, it is far from a magic hormone balance solution. Soy contains compounds that block the absorption of needed nutrients like zinc and will disable enzymes your body needs to access other nutrients. It directly blocks thyroid function and protein absorption. Many people are allergic to soy products, and women who are extremely sensitive to estrogens of any kind may react negatively to them.

The traditional Asian processing methods used to make fermented soy products--tofu, tempeh, and miso—get rid of most of the toxins and make the beneficial phytochemicals more available in the body. Tofu and tempeh are a nearly complete protein and as such are an excellent alternative to meat in a balanced meal. Miso stirred into hot water with a strip of kombu or nori (seaweeds) makes a satisfying soup base or beverage. To offset the negative side of soy, Dr. David Zava recommends eating fermented soy products and tofu as the Asians do, with a protein such as fish and a rich mineral source such as the sea-weeds.

Soy milks and soy protein powders aren't in the same league as the fermented soy products, so use them sparingly. There's a good chance that the soybean toxins are more concentrated in these products, and they may do you more harm than good over the long haul.

Please don't eat soy three times a day or even every day. That undermines your goal of balance. Aim for two or three times a week and get the rest of your phytochemicals from a variety of fresh fruits and vegetables."

Health Hazards of Soy

1. High levels of phytic acid in soy reduce assimilation of calcium, magnesium, copper, iron and zinc. Phytic acid in soy is not neutralised by ordinary preparation methods such as soaking, sprouting and long, slow cooking. High phytate diets have caused growth problems in children.
2. Trypsin inhibitors in soy interfere with protein digestion and may cause pancreatic disorders. In test animals soy containing trypsin inhibitors caused stunted growth.
3. Soy phytoestrogens disrupt endocrine function and have the potential to cause infertility and to promote breast cancer in adult women.
4. Soy phytoestrogens are potent anti-thyroid agents that cause hypothyroidism and may cause thyroid cancer. In infants, consumption of soy formula has been linked to autoimmune thyroid disease.
5. Vitamin B12 analogs in soy are not absorbed and actually increase the body's requirement for B12.
6. Soy foods increase the body's requirement for vitamin D.
7. Fragile proteins are denatured during high temperature processing to make soy protein isolate and textured vegetable protein.
8. Processing of soy protein results in the formation of toxic lysinoalanine and highly carcinogenic nitrosamines.
9. Free glutamic acid or MSG, a potent neurotoxin, is formed during soy food processing

and additional amounts are added to many soy foods.

10. Soy foods contain high levels of aluminium which is toxic to the nervous system and the kidneys

11. The various negative effects of soy weaken the immune system.

Phytic Acid and Soy

Phytic acid is a part of the soy bean's makeup which is found in the husk of the bean – and also totally destroys the credibility of the manufacturers' claims that soy products are a good source of calcium and help prevent osteoporosis. Because soy contains more phytic acid than any other grain or pulse, and because phytic acid impairs absorption of most minerals, especially calcium, soy actually strips your body of calcium.

Although not a household word, phytic acid has been extensively studied; there are literally hundreds of articles on the effects of phytic acid in the current scientific literature. Scientists are in general agreement that grain - and legume-based diets high in phytates contribute to widespread mineral deficiencies in third world countries.

The soybean has one of the highest phytate levels of any grain or legume that has been studied, and the phytates in soy are highly resistant to normal phytate-reducing techniques such as long, slow cooking. Only a long period of fermentation will significantly reduce the phytate content of soybeans.

Phytic acid has been highlighted by Dian Mills in her book 'Endometriosis - Healing through Diet and Nutrition', as being a particular compound that is found in wheat. She speculates that it is the phytic acid in wheat which aggravates the symptoms of endometriosis. Phytic acid is found at higher levels in soy than it is in wheat, but many women who use a diet for endometriosis are substituting their dairy and protein intake with soy products. This will obviously negate the benefits of a targeted diet for endometriosis.

GM Crop

Most soybeans are grown on farms that use toxic pesticides and herbicides, and many are from genetically engineered plants. When you consider that two-thirds of all manufactured food products contain some form of soy, it becomes clear just how many Americans are consuming GM products, whose long-term effects are completely unknown

PR and Soy

The public relations machine extolling the virtues of soy has been global and relentless. It has to be - there are at least 100 million acres of soy under cultivation in the United States alone, much of it genetically engineered.

The Monsanto Corporation has 45 million acres of genetically modified soybeans growing in the United States. American law permits these crops to be mixed with a small amount of organic soybeans, and the resultant combination may then be **labelled organic!**

It is not only the media who bear responsibility for helping the soy industry carry out this mass-manipulation and brainwashing of the public. Many health professionals are so busy, and probably totally unaware of the truth about Soy, that they are unable to counsel and advise their patients correctly regarding diet.

Consider the words of Dr Raymond Peat, the noted endocrine physiologist at the University of Oregon who was one of the first to blow the whistle on the dangers of HRT, years before it finally made headlines:

"There is a distinct herd instinct among people who 'work in science' which makes it easy to believe whatever sounds plausible, if a lot of other people are saying it is true. Sometimes powerful economic interests help people to change their beliefs. For example, two of the biggest industries in the world, the estrogen industry and the soy bean industry, spend vast amounts of money helping people to believe certain plausible-sounding things that help them sell their products."

You are going to come across many sources of advice and information about soy, which will extol the wonderful virtues of this protein substitute. This advice will, without exception come from the PR machine of the soy growers. Research this subject further for yourself.

This statement comes from the home page of a web site that provides informed information about soy:

'Uncovering the Truth about Soy'

'Have you ever wondered about soy? It's promoted as the miracle food that will feed the world while at the same time prevent and cure all manner of diseases. But what if all you've read about soy is nothing but a multi-million dollar marketing strategy, based on scanty facts, half-truths and lies.

How could anyone get away with that? The soy industry is one of the world's most wealthy and powerful and one that will steam-roll anybody that dares suggest there may be problems with the darling soy. When we first questioned the safety of soy, representatives of Protein Technologies told us that they had:

"Teams of lawyers to crush dissenters, could buy scientists to give evidence, owned television channels and newspapers, could divert medical schools and could even influence governments".'

The information on their web site is very revealing and is well worth checking out. You can find them at: www.soyonlineservice.co.nz

Soy testimonial

'I was looking into hypothyroidism and came across info that led me to you. My 'story' really isn't about my thyroid, but about how my menstrual cycle was altered by eating roasted soybeans. You see, I'm allergic to peanuts, and a few years back, I thought I was in heaven when I discovered these soybeans. I must say I ate quite a few over a few-week period, and then I got two periods 14 days apart instead of the usual 25 or 26 days. I visited my General Practitioner, who is a pretty smart lady, and she figured that the soybeans had disrupted my cycles, due to the high levels of phytosterols in them. I was very disappointed that I couldn't eat soybeans as well as peanuts, and tried them again a few months later. The very same thing happened to my menstrual cycle again, and that convinced me that the soybeans were to blame. My cycle has always been very regular, so that's how I knew something was going on. Also, my breasts were extremely tender for weeks at a time after eating the soy, which supported the hormone disruption theory. It's funny, because I've always wondered about the effects on the general population of eating soy products. I didn't think I could be the only one affected. Kinda makes me wonder about how I got hypothyroidism after a few years on a meatless diet, but not able to eat nuts or whole grains (allergic to those too!). So, I discovered tofu, which I like, and ate quite a bit of. Now I eat animal protein and take Synthroid, and feel better than I have in years.'

Many women who change their old diet for a diet to control endometriosis will be replacing the dairy and protein foods and substituting them with soy products. These will include soy milk, soy spreads, soy cheeses, soy based burgers and substitute meats, and many other alternative soy products.

You need to avoid all modern soy based foods and food substitutes. The only safe soy foods are those that come from eastern traditions of fermented foods like miso, tempeh and tamari. These foods are safe enough for the healthy person, but for women with endometriosis their consumption needs to be minimal because of the high levels of phytoestrogens.

There are thousands of recipe books loaded with so-called healthy meat alternatives, and 9 times out of 10 this includes alternative soy based products. People will be of the belief that their meat free, dairy free diet is safe and healthy, when in fact the opposite is true. This is why I had to trawl far and wide to find recipes for my other book, 'Recipes for the Endometriosis Diet' which were suitable, or adapting the recipe by removing the soy based ingredient or finding an alternative.

Sprouts for Goodness

Sprouted seeds and grains are simply packed with nutrients, vitamins and minerals. The vitamin content of seeds increases dramatically when they geminate. The vitamin B2 in an oat grain rises by 1300 per cent almost as soon as the seed sprouts, and by the time tiny leaves are formed, it has risen by 2000 per cent. Some sprouted seeds and grains are believed to have anti-cancer properties.

Another attractive thing about sprouts is their price. The basic seeds and grains are cheap and readily available in supermarkets and health stores - chickpeas, brown lentils, mung beans, wheat grains, alfalfa etc. You sprout them yourself, and all you have to add is fresh water. You then have easily accessible, organically grown fresh vegetables that are full of nutrients.

Sprouting is easily done, and once germinated can be kept in the fridge in polythene bags for up to a week. Most people grow sprouts in glass jars covered with nylon mesh held in place with and elastic band around the neck. You can also buy special sprouting containers from health-shops.

As well as the nutritional benefits of eating sprouted seeds and pulses, the others benefits are that you can feed yourself very cheaply by sprouting them yourself, and you can be confident that you are eating organic food. By eating a mixture of different sprouted seeds and pulses you can provide your body with all the vital nutrients and minerals your body needs.

Water

When it comes to regeneration and rejuvenating the body, water is the most important nutrient of all. When you become dehydrated the chemical reactions in your cells become sluggish. Also your body cannot build new tissue effectively, toxic products build up in your blood-stream, your blood volume decreases and less oxygen and fewer nutrients are transported to your cells. Dehydration also results making you feel weak and tired.

The brain is seventy-five per cent water, this is why the quantity and quality of water you drink also affects how you feel and think. For mental clarity and emotional balance you need plenty of water. Drinking enough also provides us with energy; it stops us from having water-retention because the body is not in a state of panic and holding onto water all the time; in turn, water assists with banishing cellulite.

So you can see the vital importance of water for our bodies to stay in balance. The quality of water you drink matters a lot. If you can afford it, then buy the best spring water. If not, then at least get yourself a good water filter and use it always, changing the filter regularly. Bottled waters differ tremendously. Some of those sold in plastic containers in the super-market are nothing more than tap water which has been run through conditioning filters to remove the taste, while doing nothing to improve the quality.

For basic good health, you need to be drinking around eight big glasses of water a day. Getting into the water habit will quench your appetite, heighten your energy levels, improve the look of your skin, as well as all the health benefits.

Some Cooking Cautionary Notes

Cooking Food

When buying and preparing food, select the best quality foods possible. Take care when storing, preparing and cooking food, that the nutrients are not damaged and toxic chemicals are not introduced. For instance, avoid preparing vegetables in advance, since they will lose their vitamins if allowed to soak for long in water.

Microwave cooking causes a loss of nutrients, but whether this is greater than in any other form of cooking is not yet known. Toasting and browning alters the chemical composition of the surface layers and may destroy amino acids and vitamins. Frying is to be avoided if possible; not only does it increase the amount of fat in the diet, but high temperatures can produce carcinogens in fats.

Utensils

Even the implements you use when cooking can affect health. Rinse detergents thoroughly from kitchenware, since experiments have linked them with eczema and damage to the intestinal lining. Earthenware pots are sometimes glazed with lead or cadmium, which can be dangerous. White porcelain or glass containers are more suitable. Copper, brass or aluminium pans should be avoided. Aluminium, especially, may be associated with digestive-system complaints ranging from mouth ulcers to piles. Aluminium in the system has also been associated with Alzheimer's disease. Non-stick Teflon coatings may lead to gut ulcers when they start to peel off.

Stainless steel pans are suitable, especially if they have the copper insert, sandwiched in the bottom, as this allows quick and even distribution of heat. Iron utensils are recommended since they distribute heat evenly for thorough cooking, and they may also be a source of iron in the diet.

Meat and Dairy

Meat, dairy and eggs promote the pro-inflammatory prostaglandins and should be avoided if possible. Modern meat rearing now involves administering hormones to animals in the form of ear implants. One of these hormones, zeranol, is a form of estrogen made from mould called fusarium. This hormone occurs naturally in crops cut in damp weather and the level of the natural hormone can be quite high. Antibiotics have also been used as a growth promoter for forty years and we now get a small but insidious dose of antibiotics in nearly every meat and dairy product we eat.

Regarding poultry eggs, they are naturally produced through the hormone process, which in turn will be based on estrogen. Cheese is made by adding rennet, which comes from calves' stomachs. Vegetable rennet is not derived from a vegetable source but from chemicals. Cows' milk is meant for feeding calves, and is not assimilated into the human digestive system very well. Goats' milk is easier to digest. Pasteurised cows milk is vastly deficient in vitamins A, B, and, calcium, iodine and the enzymes that make it more digestible.

In addition, a large percentage of women are noticeably zinc-deficient and some animals ingest copper-containing formulae which makes this balance even worse because copper is antagonistic to zinc. Copper also keeps estrogen levels high. Interestingly, copper is used in birth control pills as copper helps control the ovulation cycle.

Coffee and Tea

The caffeine in coffee is linked to heart disease, and coffee drinkers suffer from 60 per cent more heart attacks than people who do not drink it. Coffee also causes palpitations, raises blood pressure and cholesterol levels, increases stomach acid secretions, aggravate fibrocystic breast disease and increases the risk of miscarriages and birth defects. Its psychological effects include insomnia, anxiety, panic attacks and depression. Decaffeinated coffee is no better. Trichloroethylene was used to decaffeinate coffee until quite recently when it was proved to be carcinogenic. Now petrol-based solvents are often used instead, which is just as worrying. The alternatives are grain coffee made from cereals and fruits and are readily available in health-food shops.

The levels of caffeine in tea are as potent as in coffee, which make it a very strong stimulant. The tannin in it curbs hunger pangs and it is so astringent that it inhibits the absorption of iron. Your alternatives are green tea from China, which has its own medicinal properties, and herbal teas. Camomile tea works wonderfully to soothe. It aids restful sleep and soothes the digestive tract.

For further advice and information about Diet and Endometriosis please refer to my other book 'Recipes for the Endometriosis Diet'. Some of the basic guidelines from this book have already been included here, but you will find even more clarification and advice along with loads of tasty recipes.

Vitamins and Minerals

Vitamins and minerals are an essential part of any diet. The best and most natural way to obtain vitamins and minerals is through food intake. Below is a run-down of the vitamins and minerals which are most needed by women with endometriosis, which your body needs to gain optimum health. If you feel that you have any particular vitamin or mineral deficiency, which cannot be obtained from your diet, then you need to take good quality Vitamin and Mineral Supplements.

For many of our nutritional needs we can change our food intake to optimise and increase the trace elements we require. But there are certain vitamins and minerals which will need to be supplemented because they are not obtainable through the food chain. This is especially so with minerals like Selenium, which should be taken up from the soil and enter the food chain from the natural growth of vegetables and grains. Today most of the soil on the planet is seriously depleted of Selenium, so supplementing this trace element is required in your diet.

Calcium

Calcium levels in menstruating women decrease 10 - 14 days before the onset of menstruation.

Deficiency may lead to headaches, muscle cramps or pelvic pain. Most sources of calcium are from dairy products, which need to be avoided by women with endometriosis. Calcium can be obtained from green tea, dried beans, green vegetables, sunflower seeds and sardines.

Magnesium

Magnesium is a mineral that is believed to ease cramping at the time of menstruation. A deficiency in magnesium may trigger muscle cramping, menstrual cramping, insomnia, and rapid heart rate. Excellent sources of magnesium are brussel sprouts, leafy green vegetables, figs, apples, almonds, nuts and seeds. Taking magnesium with calcium in supplements such as dolomite, aids the absorption of both minerals. This is one of the key minerals, which when supplemented by women who have endometriosis, have had good results with relieving their symptoms.

Zinc

Zinc is one of the controlling nutrients for progesterone production. It is essential for enzyme activity, helping cells to reproduce. It is thought that deficiencies in zinc affect the immune system and resistance to infection by weakening the white blood cells. Supplementation with zinc will help women better cope emotionally with menstruation, and eliminate some of the irritability that can accompany the monthly cycle. Also, it boosts the immune system. Good sources include shellfish, nuts and whole grain cereals.

Iron

Women loose about 30mg of iron per menstrual period. However, some women with endometriosis have very heavy periods, and may loose substantially more iron. These women are at risk of iron deficiency anaemia, which is characterised by weakness, extreme fatigue and mental fog. When taking iron supplements, they should be divided with two meals for better absorption. Most of the dietary sources of iron are to be found in foods that are best avoided by women with endometriosis, so a supplement is advised.

Potassium

Potassium is essential for muscle contraction, regulation of heart rate, conduction of nerve impulses and fluid balance in the body. Many women may become deficient in potassium due to bouts of diarrhoea during the menstrual cycle, and have bloating, weakness and fatigue. Some good sources of potassium are bananas, apricots, oranges, potatoes and dark green leafy vegetables.

B Vitamins

The B vitamins are all involved in the breakdown of proteins, carbohydrates and fats in the body. If there is a deficiency in either B12 or folic acid, anaemia may occur. It is important to take a B-complex vitamin at meal times, as the stomach is full and the side-effects of nausea can be offset. Excellent sources of B vitamins include dark leafy greens, whole grains, oatmeal, lima beans, tuna, and asparagus. Overcooking, canning, long-term storage of vegetables can decrease the B vitamins in food, so they are best eaten when they are fresh.

Vitamin C

Vitamin C is instrumental in building and maintaining collagen within the body; it strengthens blood vessel walls and aids absorption of iron. It can also promote healing after surgery. It is thought to stimulate the immune system to promote healing and provide resistance to disease. Sources include brussel sprouts, green/red peppers, kale.

Vitamin A

Vitamin A is found in yellow, red, orange, or dark green leafy vegetables. It is proposed that it works as an immune system booster. It is recommended by some to help prevent thick scar formation and to maintain healthy skin. Vitamin E is also advised if you have fertility problems. If you have high blood pressure and are on anticoagulant drugs, check with your doctor before taking vitamin E as a supplement.

Additional Supplements Specifically to Deal With Endometriosis

Some of these supplements are not so well known but are proving to be of benefit for women with endometriosis.

Selenium

Selenium is an important mineral for women with endometriosis because of its anti-inflammatory properties. As mentioned earlier, we can easily become deficient in this mineral because the main way to get it into our systems is through plant foods, which take up selenium from the soil, or from livestock that absorbs it from their own food supply. Over years of intensive farming and soil depletion, selenium is becoming more scarce in the food chain.

Interestingly, in cattle, endometriosis can be due to selenium deficiency. So farmers supplement their cattle with selenium along with other vital nutrients in the form of a salt lick. Farmers must have fit healthy cattle that breed, otherwise they are out of business; a herd with endometriosis would mean bankruptcy.

Selenium is needed in every cell of our bodies, and is in particularly high concentrations in the kidneys, liver, pancreas, spleen, and testes.

The most concentrated food source for selenium is the Brazil nut; a single one contains 120 mcg, (which is about twice the RDA). Seafood in general, as well as poultry and meat, are also good sources. So are grains, especially oats and brown rice.

The concentration of selenium in all these food sources depends on a variable that's very hard for people to determine: the level of selenium in the soil in which the plant grew (and which the animal then ate). Only in the past two decades have scientists begun to understand just what a vital role selenium plays in numerous biological functions. Perhaps its most crucial job is to prevent disease.

Health Benefits of Selenium

Selenium has many tasks to perform in the body. It helps to boost the immune system and fight off infection, providing a general increase in the body's defence against dangerous bacteria, viruses, and cancer cells. On a basic cellular level, every cell in the body needs a particular hormone from the thyroid gland that selenium helps to convert to an active form.

Perhaps the most famed use of selenium in supplement form is as an antioxidant; it helps to mop up dangerous molecules known as free radicals that can damage and alter healthy cells. It has also been recommended for staving off the effects of ageing.

Selenium can help with many health issues including:

Prevention of cancer. Test-tube studies indicate that in addition to fostering healthy cell growth and division, selenium discourages the formation of tumours.

When researchers at Cornell University and the University of Arizona pooled results from 5-year studies designed to assess the effects of selenium supplements (200 mcg daily), they came up with some startling findings: Compared with the rest of the population, participants had 63% fewer prostate cancers, 58% fewer colorectal tumours, and 46% fewer lung cancers. Overall, their death rate from cancer was 39% lower than the average.

Protect against heart attack and stroke. Selenium may decrease the "stickiness" of the blood, lessening its tendency to clot and thus reducing the risk of heart attack and stroke. In addition, the mineral may encourage healthy heart function by increasing the proportion of HDL ("good") cholesterol to LDL ("bad") cholesterol. People who have already had a heart attack or a stroke, or who smoke, appear to benefit the most from selenium.

Anti-inflammatory properties. Selenium's antioxidant and anti-inflammatory actions may be enhanced when combined with vitamin E. For women with endometriosis, which appears to be an inflammatory auto-immune disease, this nutrient duo may foster healing of the skin and help protect the heart, blood vessels, skin, joints, and other parts of the body prone to inflammation.

Symptoms of selenium deficiency include muscle weakness and fatigue. Poor selenium intake over time may even increase the risk for cancer, immune-system problems, heart disease, and various inflammatory conditions (especially skin-related ones).

Evening Primrose Oil

Evening Primrose Oil has proved very beneficial for endometriosis sufferers as well as for women who suffer PMS.

Native to North America, the evening primrose is a tiny and short-lived wildflower and not a true primrose. When Europeans found it and took it to Europe, its purported healing properties for skin diseases and flesh wounds quickly earned it the name "King's cure-all." Evening primrose is now grown in 30 or more countries, and the oil pressed from its seed is marketed as a nutritional supplement and indeed as a miracle drug.

Essential Fatty Acids and Evening Primrose Oil

Like other nuts, seeds, and fruits (including olives, rape-seed, corn, and so forth), evening primrose seeds contain some vitamin E, and in addition, what are known as essential fatty acids (EFAs)-so called because the body needs them in order to function properly, but does not produce them. We have to consume them. The chief EFAs are linoleic acid and linoleic acid, both of which are plentiful in foods.

Evening primrose oil, however, is a source not only of linoleic acid but also of another kind of fatty acid called gamo-lenic acid (also known as gamma linoleic acid, or GLA). This fatty acid, normally manufactured by the body from linoleic acid, is important in many ways. It is transformed by the body into hormone-like chemicals that include the prostaglandins. These are the 'good' prostaglandins that help deal with the 'bad' ones. Also these good prostaglandins control such processes as inflammation, blood clotting, and cholesterol synthesis.

Agnus Castus

The berries of this plant have a range of medicinal actions but possibly the most important is its ability to rectify hormonal imbalances caused by an excess of estrogen and insufficiency of progesterone. It acts upon the pituitary gland, reducing the production of certain hormones (the ones we do not want, which are overactive) and increase the production of others (which are under-active), shifting the balance.

Thus it has a wide application of uses in malfunctions of the feminine reproductive system and has been used with great effect in restoring absent menstruation, regulating heavy periods, restoring fertility when this is caused by hormonal imbalance, relieving pre-menstrual tension and easing the change of the menopause.

Agnus Castus is also known as the Chastetree, and has been used for centuries in different parts of the world to relieve reproductive disorders. Agnus Castus is helpful in dealing with mood-swings, depression; for menopausal women it helps with hot flushes and increases libido.

For women with Endometriosis - Agnus Castus has the following benefits:

- research in Germany has shown that the berry can stimulate progesterone synthesis and secretion and balance the excess estrogen in the system
- it can regulate periods and help with the cramping and pain of endometriosis
- ease constipation and digestive problems which are so common among endometriosis sufferers. A sluggish digestion is no match for Agnus Castus

Agnus Castus has profound but subtle effects on the body and psyche, but this takes time. An improvement can be expected after eight to twelve weeks of daily use. After about a year to eighteen months you will probably find that you no longer need to use it.

I have used this herbal supplement myself, and it does work. Over time my mood is lifted and I can feel that my hormones become more balanced.

Progesterone Cream for the Treatment of Endometriosis

There are increasing numbers of women using Natural Progesterone Cream to help treat endometriosis. This treatment regime is also gaining popularity among the medical profession to help reduce symptoms and aid treatment of endometriosis.

The key ways in which Natural Progesterone Cream will help Endometriosis includes:

- Taking a high enough dose to induce a psuedo-pregnancy - this will stop the further development of endometriosis. Using Natural Progesterone Cream is a safer method to induce pseudo-pregnancy than using the synthetic Progetins that do the same thing
- Reduce further proliferation of endometriosis implants and allow any implants that are present to shrink
- Counteract estrogen dominance

Using Natural Progesterone Cream to Treat Endometriosis

Progesterone stops further development of endometrial cells. It is advised to use the cream from day 6 of the cycle to day 26 each month, using one ounce of cream per week for three weeks, and then stopping just before your expected period.

After 4 to 6 months of using the cream, women are reporting that their menstrual pains gradually subside as monthly bleeding from the endometriosis implants becomes less and healing of the inflammatory sites starts to occur.

Natural progesterone is **not** the same as progestin in prescription birth control pills, or the progestin used in the treatment of endometriosis. These prescription hormones are chemically modified from the natural hormones to be different in order to be patented. This then allows pharmaceutical companies to manufacture these chemically based hormones for profit.

Since these chemically modified hormones are not naturally found in nature or in the body, they have many potentially dangerous side effects. In contrast, natural progesterone is bio-identical to the hormone in your body, and is compatible with the human body with a minimal amount of side effects.

Please note: You must make sure to avoid xenoestrogens. If you do NOT avoid xenoestrogens and take natural progesterone, the endometriosis may worsen. This is because the natural progesterone re-sensitises the estrogen receptors back to normal. Long term chronic xenoestrogen exposure causes the estrogen sensors to be desensitised.

Do Not Use Progestins with Progesterone

Synthetic Progestins such as Megestrol and Provera compete with the receptor/binding sites normally reserved for Progesterone. Progesterone taken together with these synthetic hormones will not work. You are advised to withdraw from using synthetic Progestins gradually before starting to use natural progesterone for the treatment of endometriosis.

How to use Progesterone Cream for the treatment of Endometriosis

- Use a progesterone cream with at least 500 mg of natural progesterone per ounce
- For 4-6 months - use between 1 ½ to 3 ounces of cream per month. Use on days 6 though 26, where day 1 is the first day of your period. This is about one half (½) or one (1) teaspoon per day. This works out to 60-70 mg/day of Natural Progesterone
- Rub the cream on any part of the body that has good circulation before bed time - beasts, neck, chest, legs, arms, thighs, soles of the feet, or back
- If you have a lot of body fat, the progesterone must be soaked up by the body fat first before getting to your body. You may need a higher dose to deal with endometriosis.

Find the Correct Progesterone Cream

Many women have thought Wild Yam extract cream and progesterone cream are the same thing. **The fact is they are not.** Many companies are marketing a cream made from wild yam extract and telling customers that their body is going to convert wild yam extract into progesterone. This is not true.

There are Progesterone creams on the market, which are being used successfully by women with Endometriosis, to help them deal with the disease, and to help with estrogen dominance. The only successful results however, are from those creams which contain a synthetic natural progesterone. This means that the progesterone being synthesised is identical to the human hormone progesterone at a molecular level. It will never be completely identical as we cannot replicate nature, but it will be as close as possible. So this 'natural progesterone' is synthetic and is made in a laboratory.

Some companies who make Wild Yam cream have even stated 'This plant makes a substance identical to the progesterone produced by the human body', which is not true. So all this misleading and deceptive information is confusing women, and they are paying a lot of money for a product that does not live up to its claims. Granted, there are some beneficial health effects from using a yam based cream, but nothing in the way of the benefits to be gained from the synthetic progesterone creams.

Scientific studies have shown time and time again that for any natural progesterone cream to really be effective and increase the progesterone levels in your blood stream, there are two important factors. Firstly, a truly effective cream must contain synthetic natural progesterone, not wild yam extract. Secondly, a truly effective cream must contain a **minimum** of 400mg of natural progesterone per ounce.

This confusion seems to have easily arisen because the synthetic natural progesterone is actually made from the Wild Mexican Yam plant extract.

Ah ha! I hear you say. So that is why it is so easy to be confused. It is the people who manufacture these creams who are at fault, obviously; not the hundreds of individuals who are selling it for them on the myriad of Internet health web-sites.

To make the synthetic natural progesterone, requires a laboratory procedure to extract the active ingredients in the Wild Yam extract, which is synthesised with the aid of an enzyme, thus turning it into a hormone. Unlike synthetic estrogen and progestin, synthetic natural progesterone is not a drug and it does not have any side effects associated with it. You can use this product knowing that it is safe.

So beware of all the hype surrounding the sale of Wild Yam creams. Do not pay attention to claims that the ingredients of these creams can covert in the body to progesterone. It has been tested and proven not to be the case. The bottom line is that you need to purchase a good quality, high dose **synthetic natural progesterone** to achieve any benefits. This is especially important for the treatment of Endometriosis.

Also be aware of any added ingredients in Natural Progesterone Cream. Some makes of cream have been found to include various Parabens, which is a group of compounds used in most toiletries, to stop the deterioration of a product. Parabens are another form of xenoestrogen, which rather defeats the object of using the cream. There are Natural Progesterone Creams available that **do not** include parabens.

So shop around, do your research, and purchase the best quality Natural Progesterone Cream, to use for the treatment of Endometriosis. These creams can be expensive and you cannot afford to be wasting your money and raising your hopes, only to find you are not getting the desired results.

Sulphur (Methyl Sulphonyl Methane - MSM)

This is one mineral that I have not seen mentioned once in any discussions regarding help for endometriosis, but it does have very obvious benefits. The main benefits are the pain relieving and anti-inflammatory properties of this supplement.

MSM is Methyl Sulphonyl Methane - is a form of organic sulphur that is stored in every cell of our bodies. The body uses sulphur continuously to create new cells; without it the body will produce weak and dysfunctional cells.

We are supposed to get sulphur from our food but even washing food can remove the sulphur; processing food certainly will. Sulphur surprisingly is the third most abundant substance in our bodies. If we do not feed ourselves enough sulphur there will be consequences and sulphur deficiencies have been associated with arthritis, acne, rashes, depression and memory loss as well as slow wound healing, gastrointestinal problems, inflammatory problems, scar tissue, lung dysfunction and immune dysfunction. As sulphur is lost in food processing, sulphur deficiencies are very common today.

What will it do?

It will make everything soft. It can soften your eyeballs making them easier for your eye muscles to focus; it can soften your digestive system making it impossible for parasites to get a grip; it can soften your hormonal glands returning them to optimal functioning; it can soften your brain making it difficult for heavy metals to get a grip; it can soften your muscles and ease muscular discomfort and tension; and within four or five days of taking an MSM supplement, it will soften your skin noticeably. This last change I can testify to, because it has softened my skin.

MSM for Pain relief and Inflammation

Approximately half of the total body sulphur is concentrated in the muscles, skin and bones. One of the most significant uses of MSM as a supplement is its demonstrated ability to relieve pain and inflammation. When rigid fibrous tissue cells swell and become inflamed, pressure and pain result. Since MSM can restore flexibility and permeability to cell walls, fluids can pass through the tissues more easily. This helps equalise pressure and reduce or eliminate the cause of pain. Harmful substances such as lactic acid and toxins are allowed to flow out, while nutrients are permitted to flow in. This prevents the pressure build-up in cells that causes inflammation.

How does MSM Work

MSM makes cell walls permeable, allowing water and nutrients to freely flow into cells and allowing wastes and toxins to properly flow out. The body uses MSM along with Vitamin C to create new, healthy cells, and MSM provides the flexible bond between the cells. Without proper levels of MSM, our bodies are unable to build good healthy cells, and this leads to problems such as lost flexibility, scar tissue, wrinkles, varicose veins, hardened arteries, damaged lung tissues, dry cracking skin, digestive disorders, joint problems, and inability to defend against allergic reactions to food, animals and plants.

MSM is an anti-oxidant that helps to clean the blood stream and flush toxins trapped in our cells. It is also a foreign protein and free radical scavenger. In order to maintain good health, we need to supplement our diets with MSM, to enable the body to heal itself. The body uses what it needs, and after 12 hours will flush out any excess amounts.

MSM is available as a supplement in a variety of forms. I have found the cheapest to be a loose powder which I mix with orange juice, and take first thing in the morning.

Feedback at endo-resolved.com after using MSM

'I recently read about MSM on your website. Having gone through Hell!!! I tried it and 3 weeks later I have had no pain!!!! It is unbelievable!! Thank you very much!!!!! Candy

Echinacea

Research has proved that Echinacea is extremely valuable for aiding the immune system, heal wounds, enhance skin, and counter infection and calm inflammation. The Sioux Indians used it for snake bites, blood poisoning and wound healing.

In Germany, researchers found that Echinacea had properties equal to and often greater than most antibiotics to prevent and heal infection. Another German study found Echinacea effective in allergy treatment because it helps prevent tissue inflammation due to harmful foreign toxins. It can boost immunity; used throughout periods of stress, it reinforces the body's defence mechanisms and heightens immunity.

As a result Echinacea is a valid support for the body, not only for the healing process, but to also ward off potential threats to the body. The properties of wound healing, heightened immunity, and prevention of tissue inflammation, are all essential aids for the body when dealing with endometriosis.

Noni Juice

Noni is a tree which grows in Polynesia. It bears fruit 365 days of the year. It is from the fruit that Noni juice is made, which has many health benefits because of its active compounds. Polynesian healers have used Noni for thousands of years for many ailments.

Noni can enhance feeling good via its ability to stimulate our bodies to produce serotonin which is known as the 'mood molecule'. Low serotonin levels in the brain are linked to clinical depression, anxiety disorders, obsessive-compulsive behaviours, bulimia, sleep problems, migraine headaches, autism, drug and alcohol addictions and patterns of violent behaviour. Raising serotonin levels can make most of these problems disappear, without have to resort to drugs like Prozac - with all its side-effects.

Other compounds found in Noni include Scopoletin which has anti-inflammatory, anti-histamine, anti-bacterial and anti-fungal properties. It also lowers blood pressure, binds to serotonin to help regulate sleep, hunger and temperature. The Anthraqunone in Noni controls infectious bacteria. The Terpenes in Noni helps with cell rejuvenation and its Phytonutrients and Selenium provide protection against free-radicals. The entire endocrine system gets a boost from Noni which has beneficial effects on the pineal gland, the thymus gland, the pancreas, adrenal glands and both male and female sex organs.

There are many testimonials on many different websites, which report on how Noni has helped people with many different illnesses, diseases and general health problems. Noni also comes in powder form which you mix with fruit juice. It is not the cheapest product, especially the juice, so the powder form is a better buy. Because of the many different beneficial actions that Noni has on the body, then it will be of obvious benefit for women with endometriosis. In fact, some women have had impressive results by using Noni juice, as well as great improvements in their overall health.

Noni is readily available in the US and Canada, and can be purchased and shipped from Hawaii if required. At the time of writing, in the UK, Noni is currently going through EEC government legislation processes, but this should be ironed out soon.

'Hello and thanks for the advice on eliminating dairy products from the diet. I also heard that there has been tremendous success with adding Noni Juice to the diet as a way to clean the system, balance hormones and eliminate pain associated with endometriosis and fibroids. I have endometriosis and have virtually eliminated the pain since using Noni Juice. I also have found that with the balancing of the hormones, my mood has improved greatly.'

From a Noni website with message board

* * *

Additional Support

Castor Oil Packs

Castor oil has been used therapeutically for hundreds of years, both internally and externally. It has been used to treat everything from colitis and peptic ulcers to arthritis and female problems from back pain to fibroids, PMS and endometriosis. Preliminary research at the George Washington School of Medicine in the US has shown that castor oil packs are likely to improve the function of the immune system. They are an excellent treatment for endometriosis, not only to alleviate discomfort but to speed recovery. You need to use them three times a week - preferably every day if time allows.

The castor oil pack is a simple procedure, yet it can produce wonderful results. They were widely used by Edgar Cayce, and American psychic, to heal many different ailments including digestive problems, Hodgkin's disease, Parkinson's disease, pelvic cellulitis, and kidney problems. Edgar Cayce suggested that castor oil packs can strengthen the Payer's Patches, which are tiny patches of lymphatic tissue in the mucosal surface of the small intestine. According to Cayce, the Payer's Patches produce substances which react with the nervous system when it reaches those areas via the blood-stream. Although the Payer's Patches were discovered in 1677, it is only recently that medical science has begun to recognise them as constituents of the body's immune system.

A double-blind study, described by Harvey Grady in a report entitled Immunomodulation through Castor Oil Packs published in a recent issue of the Journal of Naturopathic Medicine, examined lymphocyte values of 36 healthy subjects before and after topical castor oil application. This study identified castor oil as an anti-toxin, and as having impact on the lymphatic system, enhancing immunological function. The study found that castor oil pack therapy of a minimum two hour duration produced an increase in the number of T-11 cells within a 24 hour period following treatment. This T-11 cell increase represents a general boost in the body's defence status, since lymphocytes actively defend the health of the body by forming antibodies against pathogens and toxins. T-cells identify and kill viruses, fungi, bacteria and cancer cells.

As a result castor oil packs have a lot going for them for endometriosis sufferers. As they boost the body's defence system, this will in turn help to boost the depleted immune system that is associated with endometriosis. Castor oil packs also help with pain and swelling as well as the detox process.

To do a castor oil pack treatment you will need:

- 2 cotton or wool flannel cloths, about 12 inches square (a piece of old sheet is fine but make sure there are no synthetics in the fabric)
- 2 plastic sheets - one to protect the bed, one smaller to wrap around the area being treated
- hot water bottle
- 150 grams (6oz) of castor oil
- bath towels
- baking soda
- hot water
- safety pins

Method

- heat the castor oil in an enamel-lined, china or glass saucepan, hot enough to put straight onto the skin with out scalding
- immerse the cloth in it and stir round with tongs, ensuring that it gets thoroughly saturated
- meanwhile cover the bed with a plastic sheet and a large towel to protect the sheets
- lift out the saturated cloth and place it over the area to be treated. For endometriosis, the cloth needs to be placed over the central abdomen area
- cover the oil saturated cloth with the other cloth, which has been soaked in hot water and rung out
- now wrap the area securely in the in the plastic, then a towel, and secure with safety pins
- lie down carefully and lay a hot water bottle on the area being treated
- leave on overnight, or at least for 2 hours
- in the morning, strip of the pack and store in a plastic bag so that it can be reused for three or four more treatments
- after taking off the pack, wash the area with water to which baking soda has been added. This is to stop any rash from developing. Do not panic if the skin turns red and blotchy. This is temporary and merely a sign of how actively the castor oil is working
- to reuse the pack, put the oil-soaked piece of cloth back in the saucepan, pour over more castor oil, and reheat the cloth.

This does sound like a fiddly process, but once you have done it a few times it becomes more straight forward. Always buy the best quality castor oil for this treatment. Try to aim to do 2 to 3 sessions of treatment on consecutive nights and then rest for a few nights. You can keep up this regime for about 3 months and then taper off to about one session a week.

It is advised not to do a castor oil pack when you are menstruating, or if you are pregnant.

Colloidal Silver

I am including information on this one, because I think you should have it in the medicine cabinet anyway. Silver is a very powerful natural antibiotic. It has been used for thousands of years in its less effective solid form, but in more recent decades it has been used in its colloidal form. The term 'colloidal' refers to a substance that consists of ultra-fine particles that do not dissolve but remain in suspension dispersed in a continuous medium. These ultra-fine particles consist of many atoms or molecules of the original material, but so small they cannot be seen by the naked eye.

The ancient Romans and Greeks found that liquids would stay fresh longer if put in silver containers. The American pioneers found that a silver dollar put in a jug of milk would delay spoilage. They also found that if they kept their silver-ware 'hidden' in their water barrel the water would not go bad.

By the turn of the 20th century, silver was regarded as a proven germ-fighter. In medicine, a solution known as Colloidal Silver was commonly used as a mainstay of antibacterial treatment. In 1910, Dr Henry Crooks, a pioneer in colloidal chemistry, wrote that :

'… certain metals, when in a colloidal state, have a highly germicide action but are quite harmless to human beings ….. no microbe is known that is not killed by this colloidal in laboratory

experiments is six minutes, and the concentration of the silver does not exceed twenty-five parts per million... '

Much later, in the 1970s, colloidal silver once again became a valued substance. Doctors at Washington University in St Louis, stumbled upon it while searching for effective treatments for burns victims, having tried many other medicines. Jim Powell reported in an article, 'Our Mightiest Germ Fighter', published in Science Digest:

'Thanks to eye-opening research, silver is emerging as a wonder of modern medicine. An antibiotic kills perhaps a half-dozen different disease organisms, but silver kills some 650. What's more, resistant strains fail to develop when using silver.'

According to Dr Becker, a biomedical researcher, *'Silver did more than kill disease causing organisms. It promoted major growth of bone and accelerated the healing of injured tissues by over 50 per cent.'* Dr Becker also discover that silver *'profoundly stimulates healing in skin and other soft tissue in a way unlike any known natural process .... And kills the most stubborn infections of all kinds.'*

Colloidal Silver Treatment

Colloidal silver is tasteless, odourless and non-stinging to sensitive tissues. It may be taken orally, as well as put on the cuts, scrapes, open sores and warts.

It may also be used as a rinse for eczema, and other skin irritations. It can be gargled for throat infections, dropped into the eyes and ears, used vaginally and anally, as well as atomised and inhaled into the nose and lungs.

Clinical Evidence

'We have had instant success with colloidal silver and immune-compromised patients. A few examples are: pink-eye infection totally resolved in less than six hour (topically); recurrent sinus infections resolved in eight days (oral ingestion); acute cuticle infections, twenty-four hours (topically). Another major area in which we has improved our clinical results is in the are of bowel detoxification. The colloidal silver has provided excellent removal of abnormal intestinal bacteria; also it has proved to be a great adjunct to our Candida albicans, Epstein Barr virus and Chronic Fatigue Syndrome protocols.' (Dr Evans M., Kansas)

How do we get silver in our body in the first place? We get silver and all minerals in the body through the food we eat. Silver gets into the food through living soil ... where living organisms in humus soil (there are billions in a handful of soil) break down the soil so plants are provided with minerals in a form to be assimilated by plants.

By assimilating the plant nutrients, the minerals are transferred in our digestive tract where our bodies utilise the organic minerals through the bloodstream to the various organs of our body. Hence, we get silver from plants. If we cannot assimilate silver for some reason, or as the tissues age, or our diet has a poor level of silver, we develop a silver deficiency and an impaired immune system.

Some Interesting used of Colloidal Silver

- Swiss biochemists are studying silver's ability to interrupt the cellular replication of HIV at various stages
- Colloidal silver water-filters are approved by the US Environment Protection Agency and also by the Swiss government for use in homes and offices
- The American space agency NASA uses silver water-purifying systems for its space shuttles; so do the Russians
- The airline companies Air France, British Airways, Canadian Pacific, Japan Air Lines,

KLM, Lufthansa, and others use silver water-filters to curtail water-borne diseases
- Japanese companies are using silver to remove cyanide and nitric oxide from the air
- Water is purified by adding one-half teaspoon per gallon, shake well, wait six minutes, shake again, wait another six minutes, then drink
- It can be used in food preservative by putting ¼ teaspoon in a quart when canning, jarring up pre-prepared foods i.e. jams, pickles etc.

You do not need to use much, so a bottle will last quite a while. It usually comes in a bottle with a dropper. Again, always buy the best quality product. The bottle I purchased had some basic instructions of usage and dosage.

So I think you should agree that having some Colloidal Silver in the house will have many uses. I have used it for gum infections with swift results. Some of the properties of colloidal silver are going to be valuable in dealing with endometriosis - improve immune system, deal with problems in the gut, help with tissue repair, to name but a few. I am sure you could think of other benefits, but we need to move on ………

A small list of some herbs useful to add to your health regime

Blue Cohosh

Blue Cohosh is mainly a female glandular herb that has strong antispasmodic properties found beneficial in the relief of cramping, muscle discomfort, uterine disorders, and menstrual irregularity. Native Americans called the herb the "Papoose Root" or "Squaw Root", because in large quantities it could induce labour or menstruation, respectively, and help regulate menstruation. It is not related to black cohosh.

Blue Cohosh is indicated in any condition where there is weakness or loss of tone of the uterus. It eases the cramps of suppressed periods and the pain associated with pelvic inflammatory disease, endometriosis or fibroids, and may also be used in false labour pain or threatened miscarriage. During labour itself, this herb eases delivery. It has a tonic effect on the uterus and fallopian tubes and increases uterine muscle tone.

Dong Quai

Dong Quai is the most important female tonic remedy in Chinese Medicine. It is used for debility and poor vitality, convalescence and tiredness in women as well as all kinds of gynaecological, menstrual, or menopausal symptoms. Dong Quai is also used to provide energy, vitality and resistance to disease and is a wonderful blood tonic, promoting its production and circulation.

It is therefore used in treating anaemia, boils, headaches, venous problems, low immunity and problems of peripheral blood flow. This plant also has a reputation as a liver tonic, protecting the liver against toxins and stimulating liver metabolism. Not recommended if nursing or pregnant unless under the guidance of a medical professional.

Motherwort

The name of this plant shows its range of uses. 'Motherwort' shows its relevance to menstrual and uterine conditions (due to its alkaloid content). It has been shown to calm palpitations and normalise heart functions in general. Recently, Motherwort extract was shown to inhibit myocardial cells, which improve several aspects of coronary health. As a nervine this herb is particularly effective in treating menstrual and uterine conditions, especially those influenced by anxiety or tension such as delayed or suppressed menstruation, menopausal changes and false labour pains.

Licorice

In China, liquorice root has been called "The Great Detoxifier." It acts on the endocrine system and the liver as an anti-hepatotoxic effective in treating hepatitis and cirrhosis. Also as an expectorant and anti-inflammatory it is useful in coughs and bronchitis. A recent study found that liquorice root actually stimulates the production of interferon, that critical chemical in the immune system that could be the key to preventing and treating many immune response deficiency diseases.

A group of Russian researchers have found that liquorice root inhibits the growth of certain tumours. It is said to be beneficial as a uterine tonic and to induce normal ovulation. Caution: Excessive and prolonged use of liquorice root can cause sodium retention and potassium depletion. Potassium supplementation (75-100mg daily) prevents this problem. Not recommended if nursing or pregnant.

Passion Flower

Passion flower is the herb of choice for insomnia; it aids the transition into a restful sleep without any 'narcotic' hangover. As an anti-spasmodic it will be helpful with menstrual cramps, and endometriosis cramping. It can also be effective in nerve pain, which is another source of pain with endometriosis, and helps with other pain such as neuralgia and the viral infection of nerves called shingles.

Peruvian Maca Root

Peruvian Maca root, or Amazon Ginseng as it is sometimes referred to, is a vegetable root or tuber, related to the potato and the Mexican Wild Yam. Maca root has been used by the native Peruvians since before the time of the Incas for both its nutritional and medicinal properties. It contains significant amounts of amino acids, complex carbohydrates, vitamins B1, B2, B12, C and E and minerals, including calcium, phosphorus, zinc, magnesium and iron. This herb has been traditionally used to increase energy, vitality, stamina and endurance in athletes, promote mental clarity, as an aphrodisiac for both men and women, for male impotence, menstrual irregularities and female hormone imbalances, including menopause. Not recommended if nursing or pregnant.

Raspberry

Raspberry tea is recommended for easing menstrual cramps and helps relax the uterus. Researcher do not know the active compound of Raspberry, but they speculate that it might be Pycnogenol (OPC). In one study, taking 200mgs of OPC daily over two cycles eliminated menstrual cramps in 60 per cent of the women who took it. Among women who took OPC for four cycles, the number who benefited was even higher - 60/80 per cent. So the longer you take it, the better it works.

Aloe Vera

Aloe Vera has historically been known for assisting the functions of the gastrointestinal tract, and for its properties of soothing, cleansing and helping the body to maintain healthy tissues. This plant has a reputation of facilitating digestion, aiding blood and lymphatic circulation, as well as kidney, liver and gall bladder functions. Aloe contains at least three anti-inflammatory fatty acids that are helpful for the stomach, small intestine and colon. It naturally alkalises digestive juices to prevent over acidity - a common cause of digestive complaints. A newly discovered compound in aloe, acemannan, is currently being studied for its ability to strengthen the immune system. Studies have shown acemannan to boost T-lymphocyte cells that aid natural resistance.

Milk Thistle

This plant is native to the Mediterranean and grows wild throughout Europe, North America and Australia. Milk Thistle has been used in Europe as a remedy for liver problems for thousands of years. Its use was recorded in the first century (AD 23-79), noting that the plant was excellent for protecting the liver. In the 19th century the Eclectics used the herb for varicose veins, menstrual difficulty, and congestion in the liver, spleen and kidneys. Milk thistle has also been taken to increase breast-milk production, stimulate the secretion of bile, and as a treatment for depression.

Milk thistle nutritionally supports the liver's ability to maintain normal liver function. It has shown positive effects in treating nearly every known form of liver disease, including cirrhosis, hepatitis, necroses, and liver damage due to drug and alcohol abuse. Milk thistle works due to its ability to inhibit the factors responsible for liver damage, coupled with the fact it stimulates production of new liver cells to replace old damaged ones.

Milk thistle has been proven to protect the liver from damage. The detrimental effects of environmental toxins, alcohol, drugs and chemotherapy may be countered with this valuable herb. The active chemical component in the herb is silybin, which functions as an antioxidant and is one of the most potent liver protective agents known. Clinical trials have proven silybin to be effective in treating chronic liver diseases and in protecting the liver from toxic chemicals.

Non-Toxic Toiletries

To avoid the toxic chemicals of commercial toiletries, it is now possible to purchase safe, chemical free products from a variety of companies in most countries.

Women are beginning to provide feed-back which validates the fact that when they stop using chemical based toiletries their health improves, and their symptoms of endometriosis start to improve as well. This is because nearly all chemical based toiletries contain parabens which have an estrogenic influence on the body. By cutting out these toxic toiletries and using natural, safer alternatives they are able to eliminate another form of estrogen from their bodies.

The range of good quality natural toiletries is increasing all the time so you should not have difficulty in purchasing them. Do check all the ingredients before you purchase, as some companies are advertising their products as being safe and free of chemicals, whereas they actually **do** contain some unwanted chemicals.

You also have the option to produce some of your own simple toiletries, which can easily be done at home in the kitchen. Most of these preparations use easy to obtain ingredients, some of which will already be in your kitchen cupboards.

Below I have included a selection of toiletries and beauty preparations for you to try, which includes skin care, hair care, bath time treats and other tips and ideas. Some of these ideas will also help you to save money.

Natural Aids for Beautiful Skin

There are many natural ingredients that have been found useful in promoting healthy and beautiful skin. Below is list of suggestions for different forms of facial skin care, many of which use ingredients readily available in your kitchen.

Lime Juice

Lime juice is an important natural aid for healthy skin.

Lime Juice Formula

1. For very oily skin.
   Squeeze lemon juice in a bowl of iced water. Splash this over the face, massage for five minutes and then wash off with water.
2. To improve a dull and greasy complexion.
   Mix half teaspoon of lime juice with one teaspoon of cucumber juice and a few drops of rose water. Apply on the face and neck and leave on for 15 minutes. Remove with water.
3. To improve a dry and rough skin.
   Take an egg yolk and mix in a few drops of lime and olive oil. Spread on the face and leave it till the skin feels dry. Wash off with ordinary water and splash on cold water.
4. To relieve tired eyes.
   Take four tablespoons each of lime juice and iced water. Saturate cotton pads in this water and place over your closed eyelids for 10 minutes.

Peach Treatment

The skin of the peach is useful in improving the complexion. Gently massage the inside of peach peelings on the face every night for a few minutes. Don't rub off the moisture afterwards. This will cleanse the skin thoroughly and free the pores. It also has an astringent action and tightens the muscle of the face slightly, thus preventing sagging tissues.

Anti-wrinkle cream

Mix a teaspoon of olive oil with an egg. Smooth over the face and neck with it. Let it remain till the skin gets dry.

To Remove The Cream:

Add a teaspoon of bicarbonate of soda to hot water. Stir. Dip a piece of cotton-wool to this mixture and use it to remove the cream.

Natural Beauty Mask

Ingredients

1 tablespoon of gram flour
¼ teaspoon orange peel powder (optional - or use an essential oil)
1 tablespoon beaten yoghurt

1 teaspoon olive oil

Mix the ingredients well and apply the paste to your face and neck. Let it remain till the skin starts feeling a little dry and then rub your face with your hands till it glows.

Wash your face first with warm water and then with cold water. This will remove all the embarrassing blemishes from the skin and make the skin soft and smooth.

To improve a dark and dull complexion

Ingredients

1 teaspoon of gram flour
pinch of turmeric powder
few drops of lime juice
½ teaspoon olive oil
½ teaspoon milk

Mix the ingredients together. Apply the mixture to your skin. Leave it on for half an hour. Wash off with water.

Cleansing Lotion

To one-fourth teaspoon of lime juice stir in one teaspoon each of milk and cucumber juice. Apply on the face and neck and wash off after 15 minutes. This lotion cleanses and purifies the pores of the skin.

Tangerine Juice Treatment

The use of orange or tangerine juice has also been found valuable for a glowing complexion.

Dip your fingers in fresh tangerine or orange juice. Apply it liberally over your face, chin, neck, and forehead.

Orange and Nut Tonic (Try not eating this one!)

Blanch and grind a couple of almonds to a paste and mix in two tablespoons of milk and one tablespoon each of carrot and orange juice. Apply thickly on face and neck and leave on for half an hour. Removes scars and blemishes from the face and makes it soft and smooth.

Tomato

Tomato, used externally, is good for improving the complexion.

Apply the pulp of a tomato liberally on the face. Leave this for an hour. Then wash off with warm water. Repeat this daily.

Tomato Lotion

To one tablespoon of tomato juice add a couple of drops of lime juice. Apply on face and remove after 15 minutes. It is very effective for shrinking enlarged pores.

Tomato Tonic

To two teaspoons of tomato juice add four tablespoons of buttermilk. Apply. Remove after half an hour. It is excellent for healing sunburn.

Cucumber

Grate or blend a cucumber. Apply this over the face, eyes and neck for 15 to 20 minutes. It is a great tonic for the facial skin. Regular use of cucumber prevents pimples, blackheads, wrinkles, and dryness of the face.

Apple Tonic

Mix one tablespoon of apple juice with one-fourth teaspoon of lime juice. Leave on for 20 minutes. Makes excellent tonic for combating oily skin.

Mint Juice

Application of fresh mint juice over the face every night cures pimples and prevents dryness of the skin. The juice can also be applied over eczema and contact dermatitis with beneficial results.

Yoghurt

Yoghurt is a very important natural beauty aid. Apply yoghurt on the face every morning. Wash it off after a few minutes with cold water. This will keep the complexion smooth, healthy and fresh. A mixture of yoghurt and lemon juice is ideal for softening hands.

A paste of lentil and yoghurt, applied as a mask, cleanses the skin and gives it a glow. Let it dry. When dried, remove it with fingertips and wash off with water. Honey, olive oil and a mixture of turmeric and sandalwood paste are all very effective in rejuvenating dry , parched skin.

Cleaning the Skin

Cleaning the skin is important as it removes the dead cells from the surface of the skin. It also will remove the dust and dirt that chokes the pores on the skin. If the dust is allowed to accumulate, it can block the pores thus blocking the secretion of the glands from coming to the top of the skin providing it the weapons it need to fight against infections, toxic agents etc. It also gives the shine or glow to the surface of the skin.

Soap and Natural Cleaners

Skin experts recommend avoiding soap because of its high pH. A high pH (alkaline) soap will dry the skin and diminish its life expectancy. The skin's surface is mildly acidic, having a pH of around 5. Most soaps are well over 7, and some as high as 10. Soaps with a high pH will not only dry the skin but also eliminate its acid mantle (coating on the surface).

You can now purchase natural soaps with a low pH level, which are produced by many companies. Some will be free of any scent for facial use; others will have natural scents for bath and shower use.

You can also make your own skin cleansers from natural products. For example, products that contain vegetable oils, such as coconut oil, and water, combine with sebum and allow it to be dissolved and rinsed away. At the same time, water dissolves dirt.

Effective skin cleansers can contain a number of different vegetable oils, including coconut, sesame, or palm oils. These are safe and effective cleansers that have a relatively low pH.

Another organic product that is useful in skin care is seaweed. The high mineral content of seaweed stimulates circulation, helps eliminate toxins imbedded in the skin, and leaves the skin feeling smooth. Sea-weeds can also strengthen the immunity and healing functions of the skin by providing the needed minerals.

Facial Scrubs

Facial scrubs help clean the surface of the skin by removing the dead skins and the dirt mechanically. It is recommended that you use a facial scrub that contains a mild abrasive. The coarseness of these abrasives vary. For example, it may contain a very fine, mild base of oatmeal or ground-up almonds. Some products may contain coarser materials such as silica or fine sand or the shells of almonds, apricots, or walnuts.

Sugar, Cinnamon and Soapwort Scrub

Scrub a small potato, leaving the skin on. Then grate the potato coarsely, adding enough brown muscavado sugar to form a paste. Add 1 tablespoon coarsely chopped soapwort leaf. Mix and spread over the face. Rub the skin with the flats of the fingers for a few minutes. Wash off with luke warm water.

Moisturisers

Water is the secret ingredient for dewy-fresh skin. Well-moisturised skin is soft and supple, reflects a healthy glow and ages less quickly. It prevents the skin from drying and chapping, thus slowing the ageing process.

Water moves through the body to the surface in a process called "trans-epidermal water loss" leaving skin pleasingly plump and firm. If your system is deficient in water, the skin's upper layers become dry and brittle. Drinking at least six glasses of water daily and eating fluid-rich fruits and vegetables help normalise dry or oily conditions, and is essential for preventing your body from robbing its necessary moisture at the expense of your skin.

In addition to internal liquid refreshment, skin requires external water replenishing. Moisturisers or humectants attract moisture to the skin's surface and hold it there. Younger skin only needs light conditioning whereas older skin needs specific nourishing treatments.

A wide variety of moisturisers are available that range from very inexpensive to very expensive. Examples are: vegetable glycerine, rose water, jojoba oil, vitamin E oils, sorbitol (derived from plants), honey, aloe vera, and iris.

Aloe vera is very good for skin care. Since ancient times, it has been used effectively to treat everything from dry skin, burns, and insect bites to skin irritations, acne, cuts, and abrasions.

Mineral oil, which is used in many skin care products, can dry the skin, block pores, and prevent it from breathing and eliminating waste.

Coconut Oil

Coconut Oil is excellent for skin care and moisturising the skin. It prevents destructive free-radical formation and provides protection against them. It can help to keep the skin from developing liver spots, and other blemishes caused by ageing and over exposure to sunlight. It helps to prevent sagging and wrinkling by keeping connective tissues strong and supple. In some cases it might even restore damaged or diseased skin. The oil is absorbed into the skin and into the cell structure of the connective tissues, limiting the damage excessive sun exposure can cause.

Essential Oils

Most moisturisers soothe and sit on the surface of the skin, but essential oils, with their fine molecular structure, work their way through from the surface to the inner dermis. This has the benefit of allowing the healing properties of essential oils to penetrate into the skin as well as the blood stream. My own oil of choice to use as a carrier oil for essential oils, is Almond oil, as it does not feel too heavy and is not expensive.

A rule of thumb for adding essential oils to a carrier oil is - 30ml of base oil with 6 drops of essential oil. You can use more than one type of essential oil per mix, but divide the number of drops so that the combined number still totals 6 drops to 30ml of base oil - you will not gain anything by making the mixture stronger and adding more essential oils.

There many health and beauty benefits by using essential oils on the skin. Lavender is a must for its multitude of beneficial properties for both health and beauty.

Different Oils for Skin Care

Fragile capillaries	Lemon, Camomile, Cypress, Lavender
Dermatitis	Sage, Camomile, Hyssop, Geranium
Eczema, dry	Juniper, Lavender, Geranium
Eczema, weeping	Juniper, Camomile, Bergamot
Mature skin	Rose, Lavender, Clary-sage, Frankincense
Inflamed	Clary-sage, Camomile, Lavender, Geranium
Dry	Camomile, Lavender, Geranium, Neroli, Sandalwood
Oily	Bergamot, Lemon, Geranium, Cypress, Cedarwood
Rejuvenating	Leon, Lavender, Melissa, Frankincense, Jasmine
Wrinkles	Lemon

You can use a mixture of oils to suit your skin type or address any skin problems. If you use an essential oil blend on your skin every night you will soon see improvements in your skin.

I used to have a small 'scar' on my face caused by a concentration of broken tiny capillaries. After using a combination of essential oils on my face every night, after about 6 months this scar disappeared.

Skin Toners

Toners are particularly useful for getting the blood up to the surface of the skin, which will help to nourish it, and for closing the pores.

Any herbal vinegar (an infusion made with vinegar instead of water) makes a good toner. Choose the herb which is suitable for your skin type (see below). Always dilute a herbal vinegar in proportions of 1:6 with mineral water and always use cider vinegar for your herbal vinegar - no other type will do.

Herbal milks (infusions made with milk instead of water) make soothing, nourishing toners for dry skins but obviously go off quickly and need to be made in small quantities. They will also need to be kept in the refrigerator.

Flower waters can also be used for toning and in this instance can be used neat. They are best purchased ready made. Lavender water, rose water, orange-flower water and witch hazel are readily available from good chemists.

Herbs for Various Skin Types

Oily Skins	Dry Skins	Combination Skins	Normal Skins
comfrey	borage	bay	apple mint
fennel (leaves and seeds)	ladies mantle	bay	apple mint
geranium	sorrel	camomile	comfrey
lavender	parsley	comfrey	cowslip
peppermint	violet	meadow-sweet	lemon balm
sage		rosemary	spearmint
yarrow			

Natural Bubble Bath Recipes

Lavender Bubble Bath

> 1 quart (4 cups) distilled water
> 1 4oz bar castille soap (humectant)(grated or flaked)
> 3 oz liquid glycerine (skin moisturiser)
> 6 drops Lavender essential oil

Mix all ingredients together. Store in a container. Use by pouring with warm running water.

Note: Castille soap is used to soften and moisturise the skin. It is made from 100% Olive Oil. Liquid glycerine is a by-product of soap making. Both of these can be found at health stores and drug stores.

Jasmine and Rose Bubble Bath

> 3 drops rose essential oil
> 3 drops jasmine essential oil
> 1 oz liquid glycerine
> 1 oz coconut oil
> 1 (4ox) bar castille soap (grated or flaked)
> 1 quart (4 cups) distilled water

Mix all ingredients together. Store in a container. Pour in running warm water.

Natural Hair Treatments

Herbal Conditioner for Dry Hair

> 1 pint boiling water
> 1 teaspoon each burdock root, calendula flowers, camomile flowers, lavender flowers
>   and rosemary leaves
> 1 tablespoon vinegar

Pour boiling water over herbs and steep for about 30 minutes. Strain and add vinegar. Pour over scalp and hair as final rinse after shampooing. Leave on without rinsing out. For dandruff, add 6 drops sage essential oil; shake well before using.

Oil Treatment for Dry Hair

> 2 ounces aloe vera gel
> 2 ounces castor oil
> 6 drops each rose geranium cedar (or sandalwood) and rosemary essential oils
> 2 drops ginger essential oil (optional)

Combine ingredients. Warm oil slightly. Comb and part hair into different sections, then massage oil into scalp. Cover head with a towel and leave it on for 1 to 2 hours, then shampoo out. Although I use castor oil because it is partially water-soluble and washes out of the hair better, other vegetable oils can also be used—the Italians have long used olive oil for hot oil treatments. In India, hot oil hair treatments are done with sesame oil, the oil of choice in traditional Indian Ayurvedic medicine, and freshly grated ginger. An easy way to add ginger to hot oil is as an essential oil.

Herbal Shampoo for Oily Hair

> 2 ounces unscented natural shampoo

10 drops lavender essential oil
2 drops camomile essential oil (optional)
Combine ingredients and shake well before shampooing.

Herbal Rinse for Oily Hair

    1 pint boiling water
    1 teaspoon each burdock root, calendula flowers, camomile flowers, lavender flowers,
        lemongrass and sage leaves
    ¼ cup vinegar

Pour boiling water over herbs and steep for about 30 minutes. Strain and add vinegar. Pour over scalp and hair as final rinse after shampooing. Leave on without rinsing out.

Soapwort Shampoo Recipe

Suitable for all hair types. Soapwort contains saponins which is similar to soap. It lathers when agitated. Lemon Verbena for a citrus fragrance and catnip to promote healthy hair growth.

    2 cups distilled water
    1½ tablespoons dried soapwort root (chopped - most health food stores will stock this)
    2 tablespoons Lemon Verbena or 2 tablespoons Catnip

Bring water to a boil add soapwort and simmer, covered for about 20 minutes. Remove from the heat, add herb then allow mixture to cool. Strain the moisture keeping the liquid. Pour into a container. Makes enough for 6 - 7 shampoos. Must be used within 8 - 10 days. Store in a cool dark place.

Lavender Vinegar Hair-rinse

Fill a one-quart jar ½ full with lavender leaves and flowers. Top with white vinegar; seal with a plastic lid, or place plastic wrap over the jar first before closing lid. Place in a dark place, such as a cupboard for 3-4 weeks. Mix one part lavender vinegar to one part distilled water and use to rinse hair after shampooing

Rosemary Hair Treatment

Use this rinse to darken, condition and tone hair.

Hot Method:

Fill a jar with fresh rosemary and cover with sunflower or almond oil. Place the jar up to the neck in a saucepan of water and bring to a medium temperature. Simmer for up to three hours. Strain through filter paper or cloth into a brown glass bottle.

Cold Method:

Follow the instructions above, except that the oil should be placed on a sunny windowsill for up to three weeks instead of heated.

The process can be repeated with the strained oil infusion and a fresh supply of herbs to make a stronger oil.

To Use:

Work the oil into the hair, then cover with plastic wrap and a warm towel. Relax in a warm place with a good book for 30 minutes to an hour, then shampoo

Beautifying your Hair

One old-fashioned, natural way to give your hair extra body is to use a setting lotion. Sixteenth and seventeenth-century herbals extol the virtues of rosemary's ability to keep hair curly. Other traditional favourites were lotions made with quince, flaxseed, gelatine, agar, Irish moss or lemon. All of these give thin hair more body and volume.

Home-made Hair Gel

Dissolve ¼ teaspoon plain gelatine in 1 cup boiling water. Let sit at room temperature until slightly set. Rub into dry or wet hair, and blow dry.

Option: Use Agar powder for the vegetarian alternative. Experiment as to the amount of Agar to use, but you will need more than for Gelatine

Natural Hair Colour

A way to perk up hair (and perk up yourself) is by changing the colour of your hair. As well as the toxic effects caused by the chemicals in modern chemical hair colours, they also do a lot of damage to the structure of the hair. Permanent hair dyes, tints and bleaches force open the hair shaft so that they can penetrate inside to alter the colour. As a result, your hair may take on the frizzy appearance associated with bleached blondes, particularly if it undergoes repeated dyeing.

Commercial natural dyes have become increasingly popular and also more sophisticated, offering a wider range of colours. Because natural hair dyes gradually fade, you do not have to worry about touching up the roots. Be sure to read the list of ingredients **carefully**, since some companies "cheat" by combining plant dyes with strong chemical dyes.

The colour variations offered by natural products are achieved by combining different herbs. Brown and amber colours are usually created by using henna combined with black walnut hull and sometimes iron oxide. For black and dark brown shades, indigo is added. Clove, sage and coffee are sometimes used in dark hair dyes. Neutral and blond henna products are not really henna at all; most often they are another herbal hair conditioner.

Camomile, calendula, turmeric and lemon can be used to increase light highlights. The basic red henna may include safflower or hibiscus to soften the colour. If you have light-coloured or grey hair, be careful when using pure henna. It may turn your hair carrot-red or a brassy orange.

Henna has been used throughout India, Egypt and the Middle East for a few thousand years to give hair a red highlight and condition it. It coats dry hair with a vegetable protein that makes it shiny with extra body, and it is drying to oily hair. (Because of this, use henna to treat dry hair no more than once every few months.) Because some people are sensitive to henna, do a patch test on your inner arm before trying this herb on your hair.

Sage and Rosemary Tea Colourant

(To restore brunette colour from grey)

Make a strong tea using dried rosemary and sage of equal amounts. Let it stand for about 15 minutes. Strain the tea and use the liquid by pouring over your head repeatedly, catching the surplus liquid in a small bowl as you pour it over your head, so you can pour it over again. Do not rinse out.

If you use this treatment regularly it will gradually change the colour of your hair and start to make the grey hairs restore back to a dark colour, but you do have to do it with every wash for at least a month to start seeing the results.

Natural Deodorant

There are alternatives to using harmful commercial deodorants. One of which is known as the Deodorant Stone.

The Deodorant Stone is reputed to be over 300% more effective than commercial deodorants. and yet it is 100% pure and natural. The Deodorant Stone does not contain any harsh chemicals, perfumes, oils, emulsified alcohol or propellants. It is made from potassium sulphate and other mineral salts which are crystallised over the period of months, then hand shaped and smoothed into the finished stone.

How it works - The Deodorant Stone is not a cover-up nor does it clog pores. The Deodorant Stone actually inhibits bacterial growth on your body. This bacterial growth is what causes body odour. So by eliminating these odour-causing bacteria it eliminates body odour. The Stone attacks the problem not the results of the problem. The Stone does not have perfume that only covers one odour with another artificial odour like some sprays or powders.

Easy to use - After bath or shower while body is still damp, simply rub the Stone to areas that need protection. (In the same manner as you would use roll-on). If your body is dry, wet the stone with water then apply.

Economical - One of these Deodorant Stones is equivalent to about 12 cans of deodorant sprays. One stone can last months, up to a year.

History - It seems that for centuries the people from the Far East have been using this pure and natural crystal as a body deodorant to help rid themselves of all body odours. The Stone is not a new-found discovery but as old as life itself.

* * *

Keeping a Diary

I personally found the process of keeping a diary which recorded my symptoms a very useful tool. I then went on to improve my record keeping and I started to keep a visual journal by plotting symptoms on graph paper.

To do this I was lucky enough to find some old ledger paper which came in large sheets, the type that used to be used by accountants. This is divided into rectangular blocks so that you have more space in each block to write or mark things down inside the blocks. I charted the 5 main symptom that I wanted to keep track of, using a column of 5 blocks, one for each symptom, and used a different colour felt pen to colour in the blocks in a different way to define what happened. I then worked along the rows, day by day, and a clear visual chart would appear. This enabled me to do a quick 'view at a glance', to see how things were going and to see what patterns in my symptoms were developing.

The main symptoms I charted were:

- days I had periods, using red felt-pen
- bowel movements, using brown felt-pen (if bowel movements were non-existent, I would leave a blank, if they were a bit light I would only colour in half the block)
- pain symptoms using purple felt-pen (if I was in a lot of pain I would colour in the

whole box, if I had average or light amount of pain, I would again, only colour in half the box)

- sleep pattern, using black felt-pen (if I slept OK I would colour in the whole box, if I slept lightly/badly I would colour in only half the box, if I hardly slept I would leave the box blank)
- energy levels, using light blue felt-pen (if I had good energy I would colour the whole box, if I had low energy I would only colour in half the box)

I also left a space at the bottom of each colour block to write in simple notes of specific events i.e. the days I took homeopathic remedies, the days I started with any supplements, days in which life had been crap, days in which life had been good, whether it was a full-moon (because I am susceptible to the full moon), appointments with the doctor/medical profession, when I was away on holiday, and so on.

Each finished sheet allowed me enough space to chart about 2 months of activity. I could then easily view how things were going and how life events were affecting my health. I could keep an accurate record of my menstrual cycle - I even put in the notes, the time of day that my period started. If I had a bad bout of Irritable Bowel, I would note down what I had eaten to give me a guide of what had triggered it off.

These visual notes can be taken to your doctor, gynaecologist or any alternative practitioner you are seeing. It is a quick, simple and concise record of all your health symptoms and is a valuable tool for them as well as yourself. I highly recommend you start to chart your health now; it may give you more clues than you realise. I kept mine pinned to the bedroom wall, above the dresser, with the pot of pens on the dresser. Using different colour pens, and colouring in the blocks, is quick and easy to do, and is much easier to read, much like an ordinary graph.

Dealing with Tiredness

This is a very common symptom with endometriosis and one that I had myself, though it was not too bad, but I did have some very bad days. This is one of the symptoms where there is not much in the way of supplements you can take to help you.

Tiredness is a key signal from your body that it is trying to deal with an imbalance in health. When we have a virus like the flu we can feel very drained. It is nature's way of making us stop, so that we rest up and let the body deal with whatever is wrong with our health. We need that energy for healing, for cell repair, wound healing, killing viruses, and to repair the body.

I do think that many of us in the West are dehydrated and we do not drink enough water. This can easily lead to fatigue. I have mentioned earlier the healing benefits of water and if we do not get enough water we start to feel sluggish and lethargic. DRINKING MORE WATER will be a good start to regaining some energy.

Many of you will be suffering from the tiredness that comes from the sheer slog, of trying to cope over a long period of time with a debilitating illness. This is natural. You need to do things that distract you, focus you, and put your concentration outside of yourself. I used to do this with gardening, and potter around for a few hours. It can be hard to do, but usually the hardest part is just starting. Once you have started then the brain chemicals kick in and you can get lost in the activity.

The more you detox your body and get rid of the toxins that are taxing your system, the quicker you will feel the benefits; gradually you will start to regain some energy. Some of the drug therapy for endometriosis can have side-effects that cause tiredness. You have the choice as to whether you continue with the drug route or whether to cleanse your system of all the drugs, toxins and junk that has been mentioned so far; you then stand a better chance to feel normal, because your body will be more normal.

Boredom can make us tired. When life puts us in a certain situation, and things becomes repetitive or dull or boring, that is when the tiredness drapes over us, like a cloud of dullness; a fog that makes us drowsy; and all we want to do is go to sleep. Even if you are not feeling up to it, go out and do something completely different - break the cycle. It may just help.

Depression can also make you feel tired, and for this you need to do lots of positive things. Depression is common amongst endometriosis sufferers, and I know why, I have been there. It is not down to one thing. It is the whole package that goes with the territory of having endometriosis. Your life feels totally out of control. So you need to do things that put you back on course. You may not go steaming ahead, but again, just starting on that course builds you up for the next stage and then the next.

Coping with Money Issues

Many of you are aware of the financial implications that endometriosis has on your life. Firstly it affects your income earning potential, as well as costing you money for treatments, supplements, books and so on.

I mentioned earlier that I managed to purchase a juice extractor by obtaining a small grant from a local trust fund. So I searched further on the subject of grants.

There are lots of grants available for individuals, for different needs, from many sources. There are grants for educational needs for those on low incomes, grants for families on low incomes and grants for the disabled. As endometriosis is a disabling disease, I was able to quantify my own grant application by classing myself disabled. I was actually in receipt of Disability Benefit at the time, which validated my application. But I feel a letter from your doctor will suffice for some grant applications.

I feel it is well worth pursuing financial assistance from these trust funds and grant bodies. Usually their forms are nowhere near as difficult or lengthy as forms from the statutory bodies. Most trust funds and grant aid organisations will not give you a lump sum to spend on on-going health care costs i.e. 6 months supply of expensive supplements. What they prefer to fund is larger single items like equipment, wheel chairs, and special adaptations in the home for disabled access.

So you could apply for:

- the juice extractor to provide you with your diet needs
- a good quality food processor to help you with your diet and special recipe preparations
- a new mattress, if yours is an old one which you can barely sleep on in comfort due to constant pain
- there are grants for disabled individuals to help them set up home-based businesses, so you could apply for financial help with additional computer equipment to do this
- there may even be some trusts who will actually finance your on-going medication/ supplement needs

Each Trust will have different criteria for grant aid and you need to target your applications accordingly. The money is there, so make use of it.

For a lot of women it is difficult to hold down a job, or maintain credibility in a job due to the amount of sick-leave they have to take. And then when they are at work they have difficulty in functioning to their full ability, due to pain, discomfort or the side-effects of drugs.

Some of these trusts have a lot of money and it I there to help people in need.

* * *

The following advice was sent to the website at Endo Resolved by Judith in Australia, to give other women some support and positive guidance - which includes 7 key suggestions to help cope with endometriosis on a day to day basis.

After reading many of your own stories, mine is pretty similar. I was first diagnosed in 1992 after reading a story about endometriosis in our local newspaper. All the previous years had been a mass of unrelated pain, misdiagnosis and so called "IBS" which was not the case. A huge jigsaw puzzle finally fitting together..! Looking back over these past 13 years, heaps of surgery and treatment, there are a few things (7)! I have learned that I would like to pass on to you all. Take the advice or not - it's up to you...!

1. If you are not comfortable with your doctor, get a referral to another, before you commit to surgery or treatment.

2. Find out as much as you can about the treatments the doctors want to give you. If you are not comfortable with the treatment and it's side effects, tell the doctor and ask for alternatives, only then can you make an informed decision. Don't be pressured into a decision on the spot.

3. Never be afraid to ask for help. There are support groups around the world who are there to help you. You are never alone and sometimes just talking to someone on the phone from the support group can be of great source of support and understanding for you or your family.

4. Always explore alternative therapies. These may include diet, natural therapies - including acupuncture, Chinese medicine, remedial massage, reflexology etc. Whilst some of you may or may not benefit from these types of alternate therapies, it is always worth a try! Never be afraid to change your diet and explore opportunities through natural medicines/therapies.

5. Never lose your sense of humor! Whilst endo may try to take up much of our time and energy and shorten our fuses a little too much, never forget to laugh. We all have our endo moments! That's what I call them... - We can look back at those kind of days- shake our heads and think "What in the hell was I thinking??? - or not thinking?" and take a laugh at ourselves. Or, Rent or go and see a funny movie and laugh a bit. It's good therapy....

6. Don't let endo consume you... There are lots more things in life than just endo. Breathing, eating, sleeping, talking, involvement with family and friends are all other things that we can do in a day. Try not to focus on the bad things, I know that's difficult if you are in pain, but try to keep busy with things that you enjoy.

7. Keep an open mind and a positive outlook. Specific treatments both mainstream medical, drug, alternate therapies etc, may not work for everyone, but keep an open mind when considering all your options. Just because it hasn't worked for one person, doesn't mean it won't for you. Give every decision you make a good run - so that you won't look back and wish you had done things differently. Try the best you can to stay positive. Looking back, knowing what I have learned over the years, there are probably many things I may have done differently - 20/20 vision in hindsight isn't really helpful at this point. Not all treatments work for all women. I know some of these seem pretty corny lines, but all have helped me get through my endo journey so far in one piece. Hope you find something that helps you too!

Other Endometriosis Healing Stories

There are growing numbers of women who have achieved various levels of healing from endometriosis. Some women have greatly improved their health to the extent that they are totally free of symptoms of this disease.

Here are a few more anecdotal stories of women who have achieved either total or partial healing of endometriosis:

Testimonial from an Acupuncturists website:

'I seemed to have had painful periods for a long as I can remember. I would be in so much pain that I knew something was wrong. I was also feeling generally unwell. I went to my doctor on and off for about 10 months, until finally I was referred to a gynaecologist. I had a Laparoscopy in the winter of 1998 and I was diagnosed with moderate to severe endometriosis. I had never heard of it before this. I was offered hormone drug treatment and was unhappy about using it. I had tried using the BCP to regulate my periods a few years before and the hormones really upset my system and I felt really ill. I decided to try acupuncture for the pain as I had read that acupuncture is good for treating pain for lots of illnesses. After 3 treatments I started to feel better. My acupuncturist said we could go further with the treatment with the purpose of boosting my immune system and hopefully to treat the endometriosis. I had regular treatments over the next 18 months and my health gradually improved as well as reducing the pain of my periods. I now have normal periods and last year I gave birth to a beautiful baby boy. I would recommend any woman to try acupuncture if they have endometriosis. I thank my acupuncturist so much.'

* * *

'My story starts when I was 17 years of age. Something was wrong, my periods were so painful because of the cramps but no one could diagnose me. The disease progressively got worse and completely debilitating and was finally diagnosed with endometriosis in 1983.

I asked the doctors what I should do, and they had no answer for me but to give me pain medication, which led to codeine, but eventually nothing could stop the pain. Incidentally, the only time I had a break from endometriosis was when I thankfully got pregnant with my daughter in 1986 but that was after four miscarriages. After I gave birth to my daughter, the endometriosis came back in two months now worse than ever before.

Finally, in 1992, I found a naturopathic doctor, who along with her husband runs one of three naturopathic schools in the United States (located in Scottsdale, AZ). I started using herbs and in one year had no more pain and am still pain free. Because of the herbs I used, I never had to have surgery, which was the next step - a hysterectomy.

My heart goes out to anyone who suffers with this. You are absolutely correct when you write how the constant pain robs you of a normal happy life. When a person has that much pain, they are miserable and irritable, such a terrible thing to endure. There had been times that I sincerely wanted to die.

Thank you for bringing some awareness to this disease.' Candy Behn.

* * *

Homeopathic Practitioner discussing the success with a woman patient who had a severe case of endometriosis:

'The second case was a 34-year-old R. N. with severe endometriosis since her teens. After four surgeries to remove large blood-filled cysts from her bladder and pelvic organs, and several courses of male hormones to suppress the condition, she came seeking only to restore her menstrual cycle, having long since abandoned any hope of childbearing. While quite painful at first, her periods had become scanty, "dead," and dark-brown as a result of so many operations and years of hormones and oral contraceptives in the past.

In the course of the treatment her menstrual flow became fuller and richer, and within six months she was pregnant. By the time I next saw her for a different ailment eight years later, she had had two healthy children after uncomplicated pregnancies and normal vaginal births, and had remained in good health ever since. While no one can attribute such an outcome to a remedy or indeed to any other agency in precise, linear fashion, my patient has never stopped thanking me for it, which is reason enough to honor and be grateful for a process by its very nature catalytic and persuasive rather than forcible or compulsory.

Furthermore, it would be a great mistake to impute these happy endings to any unusual skill of mine, since they are entirely comparable to what every experienced prescriber has seen or could easily duplicate, and I could just as well cite other patients whose conditions were far from hopeless, who believed in the remedies and In me, but whom for whatever reason I was unable to help.

Finally, I am deeply grateful that homeopathic remedies are available without prescription, and that the knowledge of how to use them is readily accessible to everyone with or without professional training. This state of affairs I take as further proof that self-healing and self-care are fundamental elements of our experience, and even a political and human right, which no government or medical bureaucracy can justly abridge or take away.'

* * *

Noni Juice testimonials:

'For several years prior to my marriage I had dealt with significant cramping prior to my menstrual cycle. Shortly after getting married seven years ago the problem escalated to the point that at times it would be severe enough to put me in bed for several days. The doctor eventually diagnosed the problem as endometriosis. The medication that was prescribed provided some relief, but the problem never really went away. My parents introduced me to Noni Juice and I started drinking a couple of ounces a day. Two weeks after started Noni, I was due for another period. To my surprise and gratitude I didn't have the usual symptoms and for the first time in a long time I had a normal experience'

* * *

'I was diagnosed with endometriosis in 1993. I was having extreme pain when I ovulated. I was having excruciating pain during my period that I would almost pass out. I would actually feel like I was delivering a baby. Sometimes I would crawl on my hand and knees just to get to the bathroom. In Nov 1993 I underwent laparoscopic surgery and was told that I would get it back. The doctor wanted me to try hormone therapy, which I definitely said 'NO'.

I started to exercise and change my diet, but it still was there. Last Oct. I started taking Noni. I would drink a bottle a week for about two months and then cut it back to a half bottle and now to about 2 to 4 oz. My symptoms started to diminish. After about 6 months it would come back, but very mild.

A friend of mine told me about supplements and superfoods. She also told me about detoxifying my intestines as well as my kidneys and bladder. I started taking the products she advised about, along with the Noni and my symptoms are gone. I feel good and along with exercising every day and changing my diet I feel like a new person. When I go for my check-ups I tell them about Noni.'

* * *

Success with homeopathy:

'After many years of unsuccessful treatments with traditional medicine and hormones I have experienced a significant change after being treated with homeopathy. I wish one of the gynaecologists or doctors would have told me before about the surprising effect homeopathy can have for women who suffer from painful periods.

I have had painful, heavy and too frequent periods all my grown-up life. I was diagnosed with endometriosis and poly-cystic ovaries many years ago. Fertility treatments (IVF) were to no avail. I have had many different treatments in the last 10 years, operations, and hormone treatments. But I continued to suffer from often extreme period pains, periods lasting 10 days and periods often every tow to three weeks.

I suffered so badly that I seriously discussed a full hysterectomy with gynaecologists and surgeons in one of the major hospitals in London. In all my years of painful periods I was treated by gynaecologists in Germany, London and New York. Although I continued to suffer from pain and too frequent, heavy periods no doctor ever mentioned homeopathy to me. Nobody told that homeopathy could have a significant and positive effect.

It was only after a friend of mine insisted that I should see a homeopath and I was still too afraid to agree to a full hysterectomy that I started to see a homeopath. She gave me the remedy 'sepia' and this profoundly changed my problems.

'After taking sepia my periods changed dramatically in a couple of months. It is now 6 months ago that I first took sepia and my periods come regularly now every four weeks. I still have some pain for the first two days, which I successfully treat with Magnesium phosphoricum (another homeopathic remedy). The rest of my period days I have no pain. I used to have pain at least 7 days and I used to take several painkillers a day during my periods before I took sepia. My period is also much shorter now than it used to be. I basically have a normal period now, it may be slightly painful but nothing compared to the painful periods I had many years before I took homeopathy.'

* * *

'After hearing my wife's gynecologist mention more Lupron shots, Gonadotrophins and a second Laparoscopy, I was desperately seeking more information on Endometriosis. That's when I bought this book. And our lives have changed for good, forever. This book led us to a doctor practising Homeopathy. After starting treatment, my wife's cyst is gone, her periods are totally painless, and guess what - she got pregnant too! Can't thank the authors enough.'

Reclaim your Life

Let's look at some of the things you can do to regain your life spiritually. This is an important part of the whole healing process. The immune system works much better when you are feeling emotionally balanced and more in control of your life.

- Do more things to get the 'feel good factor' in your life
- push yourself through the apathy barrier caused by depression - make yourself do something i.e. a bit of gardening, telephone friends, clear out your wardrobe, tidy your computer system, sort your old photos, whatever. You may feel a bit rough or tired afterwards, but you will get a buzz because you have achieved something - no matter how small it is. As long as you have made the effort.
- Get involved in activities that are absorbing, that really hold your interest. Grab the opportunity to get 'out of yourself'; a chance to stop focusing on endometriosis.
- When we are really engrossed in an activity, something we are really absorbed in and enjoy, we produce the same brain wave patterns as when we meditate. This is good for the immune system.
- Be selfish for the sake of your healing. Do not obey the demands of others all the time
- Take time out to have a laugh, this also boosts the immune system. Take out a few Marx Brothers movies or your favourite comedy videos, curl up on the couch with some (healthy) treats to nibble.
- Do get informed about endometriosis but do not get lost in the quagmire of medical information. You could start to depress yourself with the amount of negative information out there
- Join endometriosis support groups, news-groups, etc. Feeling that you are not alone in this, goes a long way to strengthening your resolve
- Do lots of positive reading about people who have fought and won against all odds, and recovered from serious illness (this helped me a lot)
- Stay focused on your goal of recovery
- Inform friends and family how you feel, and let them know your needs - they are not psychic, so they need telling

The Main Factors to Fighting Endometriosis

- **Boost your Immune System** - do everything in your power to boost your immune system. Remember your immune system is eaves dropping on you; it is listening to your emotions. As I said earlier, laughter is good for the immune system, even when you fake a laugh, it still works. Also breathe deeper.
- **Get your hormones in balance** - detox from all the bad hormones - use castor oil packs, detox diet, use a diet for Endometriosis, change your cosmetics, drink lots of healthy water, use natural progesterone cream
- **Put good stuff into your system** - organic food, diet changes, supplements, more water, more laughter
- **Take more care of your own health** - do not always leave it up to others, that is giving them the power, and taking it from you. Leaving it up to others will enforce your feelings of powerlessness.
- **Seek out support in whatever form that takes** - if you can afford it, work with an Alternative Health Practitioner of your choice who will assist you on your healing path. Read positive and informative books, join endometriosis support groups, Internet support/forums, ask friends and family for support.
- **Maintain a positive attitude that you 'will get rid of endometriosis'** - a positive attitude goes a long way towards supporting the healing process.
- **Fight back, get angry, get even**
- **Listen to your body, it has much to tell you**

There many 'ways' to heal yourself. The ultimate healing energy comes from your internal 'knowing' that you are the healer; that you are doing something to make changes. Whatever that 'something' is, be it herbalism, diet, supplements, yoga, whatever. The action you are taking and its effects on you sub-conscience will 'seep' through to your entire system and bring benefits and rewards.

There is so much you can do for yourself, you are not powerless. You can see from the healing testimonies here in this book, and on my website, that these women all had support in one form or another.

I strongly advise that you do get additional outside support from an alternative health practitioner, and one that feels right for you. You will gain emotional support as well as practical health support. You will get the impetus and assistance to stay focused on your healing. I do not think I could have succeeded with my own healing, without the support given by homeopathic treatment and the 'human' support given me by Julia, my homeopath.

There is no 'one size fits all' Remedy for this Disease

Some of you may have been hoping that this book would be the equivalent of a manual of 'How to Heal from Endometriosis'. Unfortunately that manual cannot be written as there is no one single approach, no single remedy, no set of basic guidelines where one size fits all.

No two women are the same; the treatment even using conventional modern medicine is not the same for two women. Every woman is different. Her symptoms will be different; the severity of disease will be different, her blood group, body type, hormone levels, stress levels, dietary intake, - everything is different as everyone is an individual. Which is why the fundamental approach to disease used by alternative practitioners is so relevant - which treats each patient as an individual?

This book is more of a map with sign-posts giving you directions to lots of sources of support - nutritional, emotional, and practical support.

A Crucial <u>Key</u> Point to your Healing!

All the way through this book I have talked about self help, alternative therapies, getting support, diet changes, helping yourself, ad infinitum ......

The last **key** point I must make regarding total healing of endometriosis is the need for you, and any alternative practitioner you see, to be realistic of what you can achieve. This disease causes physical damage to the internal organs, so how do you resolve this dilemma?

Don't panic, I am not going back on my claims of your ability to heal. As I keep saying, your body does the healing for you with a vibrant immune system. You support your immune system with lots of things we have covered here, and an alternative health practitioner will support you even more.

The realistic element here is that <u>not one</u> of the alternative health practises, or any supplements you take, or any dietary changes you make will undo any physical damage that has been done to the inside of your abdomen. It is possible to get success and shrink the cysts, but you will not be able to fully repair scar damage, or undo any adhesions in your abdomen. (Having said that, the supplement of MSM (sulphur) does help to soften scar tissue over time.)

There is not one homeopathic remedy, or one herbal remedy, or anything you take that can undo physical damage. There is only one answer - and that is to have surgery performed by a competent surgeon who can undo the physical damage. In most cases this can be done during a laparoscopy. The chances that you will need surgery are difficult to ascertain, because when this disease goes into remission the pain will disappear, so you will not have any evidence of what has happened to your insides.

You may still have some pains which will be caused by old adhesions, scar tissue, or by organs stuck together. This is the damage you need to get repaired. For women wishing to have children, there could be physical damage that is interfering with conception, so again, surgery will be needed in order to bring the anatomy of the reproductive organs back to as normal as possible.

Your job is to ensure that the disease goes into remission so that once you have the surgery done, it will be the final part of your healing. This is the course that my own healing took. I had 4 years of homeopathy followed by a laparoscopy where any residual scar damage and adhesions were cleared up, along with the small final cyst I had on my ovary. But do not forget what the surgeon said to me ...'that all the **active** endometriosis had dried up'

I also need to emphasise the importance of aiming to get this disease in remission before surgery, otherwise you will end up in the same position as many women who have tried to get rid of the disease by having a hysterectomy. Many women have sadly gone to the extremes of having a total hysterectomy to try and get rid of endometriosis, only to find that a few months down the road the disease comes back again. This is usually because microscopic particles of the disease were left behind in the woman's abdomen. Many factors can trigger the disease again if any amount of active endometrial tissue is left behind.

How will you know you have succeeded to get endometriosis into remission? When do you know you are ready to have surgery to repair the damage? This is difficult to answer, but in my own case I had a strong intuitive knowing that the time was right for surgery, despite having no symptoms whatsoever. Of course, not every woman will need surgery, because the physical damage may have been minimal and has not impeded on the functions of her abdominal organs. Every woman will be different. The bottom line is to not expect self-healing to repair physical damage for those of you who have had moderate to severe endometriosis.

What you can achieve is stopping this disease in its tracks and getting your whole body into steady and gradual improvement and you will feel your vitality, energy and well-being coming back to normal. The pain caused by endometriosis will disappear when you start to heal. I have had women writing to me telling me that after only one month on a controlled diet for endometriosis, their pain symptoms have disappeared. The inflammation will go down when you start to heal. The cysts will shrink when you start to heal. So some repair work does happen when you heal naturally, but only surgery will repair any serious damage that has been done by this disease.

* * *

To Summarise my Message
(At the risk of repeating myself)

Since I started my research, I have been reading so many desperate stories of women whose lives have been totally devastated by this disease. One woman had actually been omitted into hospital over 100 times. Women are cancelling entire chunks of their lives because of this disease. Many women are opting for a total hysterectomy in a last ditch attempt to gain relief from this disease. Millions of women are in despair of gaining any relief from the pain and agony associated with endometriosis, never mind hoping to be cured or healed.

Which is why I have given a candid insight into my own story - to give women hope and to spread the word that a 'cure', healing, remission, whatever you want to call it, can and does happen. There may be a few long-term successes for women who choose conventional drugs and surgery to treat their endometriosis, but they are few and far between. The best successes which are permanent are for those women who use natural and alternative treatments.

This is because using natural therapies are natural, and they enable your own body to do the healing by using your immune system to full force. Alternative therapies help you do this by strengthening your immune system. There is not one alternative therapy that does the healing for you - what they all do, without exception, is to help you to heal yourself. Ask any alternative health practitioner, and they will confirm this statement.

It does not matter if you use Homeopathy, Herbalism, Traditional Chinese Medicine, Acupuncture or whatever - they all work to the same basic 'principle'; that healing comes from within, and any alternative therapy helps the patient to help themselves.

Deciding which alternative therapy to use is down to personal choice with a mixture of finding a practitioner you 'click with', combined with a therapy that suits you. For example, if you do not like needles then Acupuncture will not be for you; if you do not like taking strong tasting concoctions, then Herbalism may not be for you. Go for the therapy which 'feels' right for you, and it will be right for you.

The other reason why alternative therapies are superior to aid healing is because they are permanent, not temporary, as in the case of drug treatment. As soon as drug treatment is stopped then the symptoms of endometriosis come rushing back with a vengeance.

I do read stories of women who have tried different alternative therapies and have felt let down. They have only felt limited benefit from the therapy they have chosen. In every story I have read of women who have 'tried' one of the alternative therapies, and have not had total success, the limiting factor has been the time span. These women have not given the therapy a chance to work. They may have only tried a regime of homeopathy or herbalism or whatever, for a few months and then given up because they were not seeing significant improvements.

My own time scale with a homeopath was 4 years - not 4 months. I was committed and determined, and my homeopath forewarned me it could take a long time to get well. But I felt that the ultimate long term benefit of total healing was far better than temporary respite. Therefore, my advice is to see any treatment using alternative therapy for endometriosis as long term (but not permanent).

People are so used to the idea of a quick fix for things in life, especially with modern medicine. We are all so impatient. But if you body has taken years to become dis-eased then it will take a long time to repair the damage and get the body back into equilibrium and balance.

To emphasise my positive message, in my research for this book and my website, I **have** found stories of other women who have successfully obtained healing from this disease. In almost every case, these women have achieved their healing through different forms of alternative treatment or diet changes or a combination of self help techniques.

The aim of my communication here is to provide hope, that there are other possibilities to gain healing of endometriosis. Evidence is mounting that it is possible, by the growing numbers of women who have achieved it.

The medical profession is not the 'be all, and end all' of health care for the human body. The medical profession is a relatively new phenomenon in the time scale of human society. Throughout history we have used herbs, healing, and essential oils. The practise of acupuncture goes back centuries; massage combined with oils goes way back in history.

Modern medicine is driven by pharmaceutical companies. There are very few doctors who develop new treatments for any of today's illnesses and diseases. It is the drugs companies who develop new treatments in the form of new drugs. And guess what, that means more profits! I admit that there have been some wonderful developments in the field of medical surgery with the use of clever, and less invasive surgical techniques, like laser surgery and fibre optics, and many lives have been saved. In turn, this includes the new surgical techniques to diagnose and treat endometriosis with Laparoscopy.

But when it comes to treating and healing diseases with drugs, then modern medicine goes in with a sledge hammer, and does more harm than good. There are the dangers of side effects, some of which are permanent and very damaging to the body; some of them even leading to death.

Your body chemistry is very delicate and the most delicate chemical system is the hormone system. We all know that endometriosis is fed and activated by hormones. In the human body, it takes only microscopic amounts of any given hormone to have a powerful and cascading effect in the body. These hormones are very potent, and yet the very treatment being offered for endometriosis by modern medicine is synthetic hormonal drugs, which will obviously throw the body into disarray and upset a finely tuned orchestra of natural chemicals in the body.

Please be kind to your body. Healing yourself is simply a matter of being committed. A total commitment to change the way you are doing things. Do not leave it up to others; take control of your own health. I did, because after I heard my treatment options from the gynaecologist, and compared that to the treatment potential using natural therapies, I knew I had no choice.

* * *

A Final Positive Word

I have lived many of the experiences you are going through. The main difference with my experiences though, is that I did not attempt any form of conventional medicine for my treatment. Granted, I did have 2 laparoscopies, but the first one was purely for diagnosis, and the second one was to finalise my treatment, as well as confirm my 'cure'.

I recognise that it must seem like an enormous task, trying to heal your own body and regain your health. After all the negative and discouraging information you have been given, trying to remain optimistic can be an up-hill struggle. But I also know, and understand, the needs and actions you need to take, which are critical to your success of achieving recovery and how to heal yourself.

All the positive steps you need to take are the ones covered in this book. None of these steps are beyond the bounds of the average woman. And do not think that you have to live a life of absolute health-focused 'mania', excluding all pleasures in life. Anyway, life is not like that. You will still have to 'live your life', doing tasks to keep your life ticking over.

My own life was fraught with stresses during my healing period. Sometimes it was like swimming in treacle! You have just read about it. Yet I still came through that maze of confusion, pain and anger; and with the help of external support, a lot of 'bloody mindedness' and a deep secure knowing that I could get well, I beat the devastating disease called endometriosis, despite all the credentials saying it was 'totally incurable'!

It could take a couple of years for you to regain your health and your life; this depends how bad the disease is in your own case. The longer you have been ill, the longer it will take to recover.   But the options of not striving for full recovery do not bare thinking about; more surgeries, more toxic drugs, more expense, more pain, recurrence of the disease, more stress, more heart-ache.

The time span to achieve success in your healing may seem rather long, especially for those who are desperate for a quick fix. Please think of this time as an investment in the rest of your life.

It is time to think outside of the box.

The more that you believe that something is going to happen; the more likely <u>it will happen</u>. This is the same with your health.   The more you believe that you will recover the more chances you have of this actually happening.

Your sub-conscious is eaves-dropping on your conscious self; so if you tell yourself, you are getting better, your sub-conscious will 'hear' that, and this message will pass on through your entire system - even to your immune system.

Looking at this from the other direction; the more negative you are, the more likely you are to stay as you are, or possibly get worse.

The saying goes 'Be careful what you ask for - you may just get it!' But if you are asking for positive things in life - then you will eventually be granted your wish, your hopes, and prayers.

It is now time to embark on your own pilgrimage towards healing. The Chinese proverb says 'The journey of a thousand miles begins with one small step.' Take this journey one step at a time, do not look back, keep your heart and mind fixed on your objective, and you will arrive at your desired destination.

With healing thoughts

Carolyn

Index

F

facial hair 73, 90
Fasting 159, 163
fatigue 7, 34, 40, 47, 49, 62, 73, 79, 84, 90, 94, 103, 167, 177, 179, 200
fibrocystic breasts 90
fibroids, uterine 90
Foetal death 85

G

geranium 134, 135, 195, 196
gestins 55, 86, 90, 96, 97, 100, 172
Gestrinone 47
GIFT 72
Ginseng 189
GnRH 46
Grad, Dr. 122
Green Tea 168, 169, 170
Growth factors 78

H

Haemoglobin 121
Hair Dye 94
hair thinning 90
Hay, Louise 29
headaches 6, 49, 90, 94, 138, 149, 162, 163, 177, 184, 188
heart disease 84
Helonias 136
herbalist 132, 133, 159
Hereditary 63, 79
high blood pressure 49
Hippocratic Oath 99
Holistic Medicine 130
Homeopathy 7, 8, 18, 72, 108, 112, 120, 136, 137, 205, 209
Hormone Disruptors 84
HRT 55, 86, 90, 97, 100, 172
hypoglycaemia 90
Hysterectomy 55
hysterectomy 43

I

Iatrogenic Transplantation Theory 79
Ibuprofen 45
Imidazolidinyl 94
Immune Deficiency Disease 80
Immune system response 78
increased blood-clotting 90
infertility 6, 33, 34, 40, 44, 51, 68, 70, 71, 72, 78, 87, 90, 100, 103, 124, 137, 171
Inflammatory response 78
Ingrid 27
insomnia 36
intercourse 35
Iron 175, 177
Irritable bowel syndrome 34

isoflavones 95, 170
Isopropyl 93, 94
IVF 71

J

jasmine 134, 135, 196

L

lavender 134, 135, 195, 196, 197
Lime juice 191
liquorice 189
Liver Disorder 79
Low sperm count 84
Lupron 48

M

Magnesium 58, 136, 177, 205
Magnesium Phosphate 136
Meditation 149
Melissa 154, 195
Menastil 155, 156
menstrual cramps 35
menstruation 36, 37, 47, 48, 63, 73, 74, 78, 81, 92, 96, 100, 150, 151, 164, 176, 177, 180, 188, 189
Milk Thistle 190
Miller, Dr. Robert 122
Miscarriage 84
miscarriage 70, 90, 188
Moss, Dr Thelma 123
Motherwort 188
MRI 41, 123
MSM 182, 183, 208
Multiple Sclerosis 29, 62, 103
Myomectomy 54

N

Nader, Ralph 100
naturopathy 29, 141
neroli 134, 135
neuralgia 189
Neurectomey 54
Noni 184, 204, 205
NSAIDs 45

O

Omega 3 28
oophorectomy 43
Oral Contraceptives 48
ovaries 42
ovary 19, 20, 27, 37, 40, 69, 70, 71, 96, 133, 208

P

pancreas 91, 168, 169, 178, 184
pancreatitis 121
Parabens 94, 182
parabens 90, 91, 94, 182, 190

Paracetamol 45
partners 4, 64
Passion flower 189
PCBs 83, 84, 85, 86, 88, 97, 168
peach 191
Pelvic Inflammatory Disease 4
Peppermint 154
Persistent Organic Pollutants 83
Peruvian Maca 189
petitgrain 135
Pfizer 101
Phytoestrogens 95, 98
placenta 70, 96
PMS 36, 90, 156, 179, 185
POPs 83, 84, 86, 97
Potassium 177, 189
pregnancy 37, 43, 44, 47, 49, 53, 69, 70, 72, 80, 82, 87, 92, 96, 133, 140, 150, 180
Primolut 47
Prince, David 86
Proctosigmoidoscopy 55
Progesterone 47, 49, 96, 98, 171, 180, 181, 182
progestins 96
Progestogen 47
Propylene Glycol 93
prostaglandins 69
Prostap 48
Provera 47
psychotherapy 148
puberty 88, 89, 96

Q
Quinn, Janet 122

R
Raspberry 110, 189
Raspberry Leaf Tea 110
rectum 42
Reiki 109, 127, 128
Renogram 55
respiratory diseases 84
rose 12, 134, 135, 191, 194, 195, 196

S
Safflower oil 165
Sage 154, 195, 198
Salpingectomy 54
Scopoletin 184
Selenium 110, 176, 178, 179, 184
Sepia 136
Shine, Betty 124
shingles 189
smallpox 136
Sodium Lauryl Sulphate 92
Soto, Dr. Ana 89
soy 95, 165, 166, 170, 171, 172, 173, 174

spermicide 89
still births 84
Sumpter, John 91
Suprecur 48
Synarel 48

T
Talc 93
tangerine 192
TCDD 86
TENS 152, 153
testicular cancer 95
Thoracentesis 55
Thyme 154
thyroid dysfunction 79, 90
Thyroid Link 79
tiredness 14, 23, 62, 64, 67, 95, 157, 188, 200, 201
T cells 78

U
ultrasound 43
United Nations 86
urine 36
uterus 54

V
vagina 42
VEGF 78, 102
Vickers, Edie 141
Voysest, Krista 138

W
Walnut oil 165
WEDO 82
Weight loss 85
West, Dr. Stanley 100
Wild Yam 181, 182, 189
Wilson, Dr. Robert 100
womb 42
Worrall, Olga 122
Wren, Barbara 29

X
Xenoestrogens 88, 98
xenoestrogens 88

Y
Yeast infections 34
ylang ylang 134, 135
Yoga 29, 30, 150, 155

Z
Zimmerman, Dr. John 122
Zinc 177
Zoladex 48

Also by the author

Recipes for the Endometriosis Diet

ISBN: 978-0-9556785-0-9
Published by Endo Resolved Dec 2007

A comprehensive diet resource for women with Endometriosis - all researched and compiled to provide a safe and healing diet to help alleviate the symptoms of endometriosis.

The book includes **over 250 recipes** plus recommendations of what to leave out of your diet and why; tips about estrogen and your diet, and how to keep it in balance; details of substitute ingredients for dairy products and baking; snippets of nutritional advice woven among the recipes; a range of recipes from simple and easy to cook through to more exotic ideas, including some recipes for parties and catering.

This is the second edition of the book, and to date there has been lots of very positive feedback from women who have followed the recipe suggestions in this book. Some women have even managed to be totally symptom free and have been able to return to normal activities in life, as well as the added benefit of loosing weight.

The purpose of the endometriosis diet is to relieve or even prevent some of the disabling symptoms that occur with menstruation, as well as the general pain of endometriosis. The diet also aims to decrease estrogen levels, stabilize hormones, increase energy levels, reduce inflammation and alleviate painful cramps.

It is anticipated that the recipes in this book will give readers ideas and guidelines of how to adapt their own favourite recipes, without jeopardising their diet regime for Endometriosis.

LaVergne, TN USA
09 December 2009

166509LV00005B/113/P

9 780955 678516